LEARNING MEDICINE

Sixteenth edition

Dedicated to the memory of Her late Majesty, Queen Elizabeth
The Queen Mother, a constant source of inspiration and strength
as Patron of St Mary's Hospital, Paddington, from 1930–2002
and of St Mary's Medical School from 1930 until its merger
with Imperial College in 1988 to form Imperial College
of Science, Technology and Medicine.

LEARNING MEDICINE

AN INFORMAL GUIDE TO A CAREER IN MEDICINE

Sixteenth edition

PETER RICHARDS MA MD PHD FRCP FMEDSCI
President, Hughes Hall, Cambridge

SIMON STOCKILL BSC MB BS DCH MRCGP
General Practitioner, London

With cartoons by Larry

and a foreword by HRH The Prince of Wales

BMJ
Books

BMJ Books is an imprint of the BMJ Publishing Group
BMA House, Tavistock Square, London WC1H 9JR
www.bmjbooks.com

First edition 1983
Second edition 1985
Third edition 1986
Fourth edition 1987
Fifth edition 1988
Sixth edition 1989
Seventh edition 1990
Eighth edition 1991
Ninth edition 1992
Tenth edition 1993
Eleventh edition 1994
Twelfth edition 1995
Thirteenth edition 1996
Fourteenth edition 1997
Fifteenth edition 2000
Sixteenth edition 2003

British Library Cataloguing in Publication Data

A catalogue record for this book is available from the British Library

ISBN 0 7279 1712 9

Typeset by SIVA Math Setters, Chennai, India
Printed and bound in Spain, by GraphyCems, Navarra

Contents

To

Spirited students, dedicated doctors, and courageous and forbearing patients—all of whom have helped us to learn medicine.

With our special thanks to all those (students of three medical schools, a patient and a BBC TV producer) who have each contributed their piece to this book—Tom Alport, Chloe-Maryse Baxter, Michael Brady, Esta Bovill, Sarah Cooper, Sarah Edwards, Adam Harrison, Farhad Islam, Liz James, Grace Robinson, Susan Spindler, Brenda Strachan—and particularly to Larry, who most generously breathed life into a "worthy cause".

I am delighted to have been invited to write the foreword to the sixteenth edition of this extremely useful guide for young people contemplating a career in medicine. The book has been written with great sensitivity and reveals the authors' deep understanding of the moral, ethical and personal dilemmas faced by today's doctors.

The Twenty-first Century presents doctors, and particularly those just embarking on a career in medicine, with new and formidable challenges. Huge advances in medical technology took place during the Twentieth Century, with the discovery of penicillin leading to subsequent generations of antibiotics and the development of transplant, replacement and keyhole surgery, to name but a few. Traditional systems of healthcare were swept aside by the adoption of a more technological approach to medicine and a view of disease focused on symptoms.

However, an increasing number of patients are now turning back to the healing methods of the past and seeking a solution to their health problems which treats the whole person and not just the individual parts. Why is this? It may be because, despite all the advances made by medical science, the answer has not been found for many common chronic conditions such as back-pain, irritable bowel syndrome, asthma, migraine and diseases such as Alzheimers, MS and cancer. It may also be that due to the very heavy workload placed on today's doctors, in part as a result of the advances made in bio-scientific medicine, they no longer have the time to develop a healing relationship with their patients. Tomorrow's doctors will need to adapt to changing needs and to develop a more integrated approach to health and healing; an approach which integrates the wisdom of the past with the scientific and technological developments of the present and the future. They will have to learn to understand and respect a variety of medical traditions and to work in partnership with practitioners whose philosophies and techniques differ very considerably from those in which they have been trained. They will need to supplement their diagnostic skills by learning from the valuable knowledge and experience of ancient traditions, such as those in India.

Recent discoveries in the field of genetic research and the human genome project fascinate, and worry, many of us. These developments have been achieved through international collaboration and hold out the possibility of new ways of identifying and treating diseases with a genetic component. However, they also raise important issues of bio-ethics, which impact on society and its values. Tomorrow's doctors will have to face difficult moral issues, which challenge both their consciences and their values.

I congratulate the authors of this very informative and useful book which, I am sure, will become essential reading.

If you choose to represent the various parts in life by holes upon a table, of different shapes—some circular, some square, some oblong—and the persons acting these parts by bits of wood of similar shapes, we shall generally find that the triangular person has got into the square hole, the oblong in the triangular, and a square person has squeezed himself into the round hole. The officer and the office, the doer and the thing done, seldom fit so exactly that we can say they were almost made for each other.

SYDNEY SMITH 1804

If we offend, it is with good will,
That you should think we come not to offend,
but with good will

A Midsummer Night's Dream
SHAKESPEARE

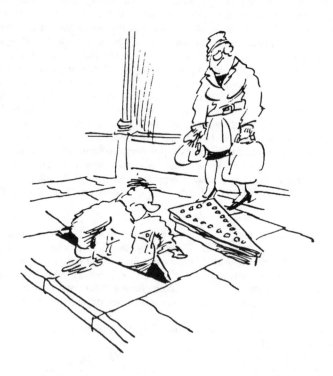

Preface

Have you read that doctors feel overworked and undervalued—that they have never been more discontented? Did you know that although doctors in training work shorter hours than ever before, their duties have never been more arduous? Have you heard that many doctors take a break after their first few posts and that not all return to medicine? Promotion is faster than it used to be, but this means that consultants find themselves doing front-line work at unsocial hours formerly done by senior trainees. General practitioners are harassed by demanding patients and submerged in paperwork. Doctors are retiring earlier—tired out, burnt out, or browned off.

On the other hand, everyone from time to time needs a caring and competent doctor—someone honest, kind, and committed to putting patients first. Most doctors enjoy doing this—most of the time. They cannot escape the reality that roses also have thorns. Medicine is not everyone's cup of tea—why should it be? If you want to be realistic about whether or not you are able to give what medicine takes, read on.

PETER RICHARDS AND SIMON STOCKILL

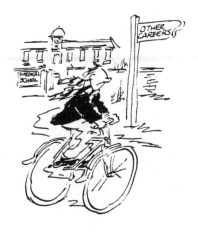

1. Why medicine and why not?

So you are thinking of becoming a doctor? But are you quite sure that you know what you are letting yourself in for? You need to look at yourself and look at the job. Working conditions and the training itself are improving, but medicine remains a harder taskmaster than most occupations. Doctors have also never been under greater pressure nor been more concerned for the future of the NHS.

Before starting medicine you really do need to think about what lies ahead. The trouble is that it is almost impossible to understand fully what the profession demands, particularly during the early years of postgraduate training, without actually doing it. Becoming a doctor is a calculated risk because it may be at least five or six years' hard grind before you begin to discover for sure whether or not you suit medicine and it suits you. And you may change; you might like it now, at your present age and in your current frame of mind, but in six years' time other pressures and priorities may have crowded into your life.

Medicine is both a university education and a professional training. The first five or six years lead to a medical degree, which becomes a licence to practise. That is followed by at least as long again in practical postgraduate training. The medical degree course at university is too long, too expensive (about £200 000 in university and NHS costs, quite apart from personal costs), and too scarce an opportunity to be used merely as an education for life.

It might seem odd not to start considering "medicine or not?" by weighing up academic credentials and chances of admission to medical school. Not so; of course academic and other attributes are necessary, but there is a real danger that bright but unsuited people, encouraged by ambitious schools, parents or their own personalities, will go for a high profile course like medicine without having considered carefully first just where it is leading. A few years later they find themselves on a conveyor belt from which it becomes increasingly difficult to step. Could inappropriate selection of students (most of whom are so gifted that they almost select themselves) account for disillusioned doctors? Think hard about the career first and consider the entry requirements afterwards.

Getting into medical school and even obtaining a degree is only the beginning of a long haul. The university course is a different ball game from the following years of general and specialist postgraduate training. Postgraduate training is physically, emotionally, and socially more demanding than the life of an undergraduate medical student on the one hand and of a settled doctor on the other. With so many uncertainties about tomorrow it is difficult to make secure and sensible decisions today. Be realistic, but do not falter simply for lack of courage; remember the words of Abraham Lincoln: "legs only have to be long enough to reach the ground".

This is your life; if you get it wrong you could become a square peg in a round hole or join the line of disillusioned dropouts. Like a submaster key, which opens both outer doors and a particular inner room, you need to fit both the necessary academic shape and also the required professional attitudes. Finally, you have to find your specific fit into one or other particular specialty.

You must have the drive and ability to acquire a medical degree, equipping you to continue to learn on the job after that. Also, you need to be able to inspire trust and to accept that the interests of the patient come before the comfort or convenience of the doctor. It also helps a lot if you are challenged and excited by clinical practice. Personality, ability, and interest, shaped and shaved during the undergraduate course and the early postgraduate years, will fit you in due course, perhaps with a bit of a squeeze, into a particular specialty "hole". Sir James Paget, a famous London surgeon in the 19th century concluded from his thirty years of experience that the major determinant of students' success as doctors was "the personal character, the very nature, the will of each student".

Why do people want to become doctors? Medicine is a popular career choice for reasons perhaps both good and not so good. And who is to say whether the reasons for going in necessarily affect the quality of what comes out?

So, why medicine?

Glamour is not a good reason; television "soaps" and novels paint a false picture. The routine, repetitive, and tiresome aspects do not receive the prominence they deserve. On the other hand, the privilege (even if an inconvenience) of being on the spot when needed, of possessing the skill to make a correct diagnosis, and having the satisfaction of explaining, reassuring, and giving appropriate treatment can be immensely fulfilling even if demanding. Yet others who do not get their kicks that way might prefer a quieter life, and there is nothing wrong with that. It is a matter of horses for courses or, to return to the analogy, well fitting pegs and holes.

An interest in how the body works in health or in disease sometimes leads to a career in medicine. Such interest might, however, be equally well served by becoming an anatomist or physiologist and undertaking a lifetime study of the structure and function of the body. As for disease itself, many scientists study aspects of disease processes without having medical qualifications. Many more people are curious about how the body works than either wish to or can become doctors. None the less, for highly able individuals medicine does, as George Eliot wrote in *Middlemarch*, present "the most perfect inter-change between science and art: offering the most direct alliance between intellectual conquest and the social good". Rightly or wrongly, it is not science itself which draws most people to medicine, but the amalgam of science and humanity.

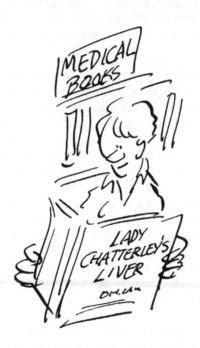

Medical diagnosis is not like attaching a car engine to a computer. Accurate assessment of the outcome of a complex web of interactions of body, mind, and environment, which is the nature of much ill health, is not achieved that way. It is a far more subjective and judgmental process. Similarly, management of ill health is not purely mechanistic. It depends on a relationship of trust, a unique passport to the minds and bodies of all kinds and conditions of men, women, and children. In return the doctor has the ethical and practical duty to work uncompromisingly for the patient's interest. That is not always straightforward. One person's best interests may conflict with another's or with the interests of society as a whole—for example, through competition for limited or highly expensive treatment. On the other side of the coin, what is possible may not in fact be in the patient's best interest—for example, resuscitation in a hopeless situation in which the patient is unable to choose for him or herself—leading to ethical dilemmas for the doctor and perhaps conflict with relatives.

Dedication to the needs of others is often given as a reason for wanting to be a doctor, but how do you either know or show you have it? Medicine has no monopoly on dedication but perhaps it is special because patients come first. As Sir Theodore Fox, for many years editor of the *Lancet*, put it:

> What is not negotiable is that our profession exists to serve the patient, whose interests come first. None but a saint could follow this principle all the time; but so many doctors have followed it so much of the time that the profession has been generally held in high regard. Whether its remedies worked or not, the public have seen medicine as a vocation, admirable because of a doctor's dedication.

A similar reason is a wish to help people, but policemen, porters, and plumbers do that too. If a more pastoral role is in mind why not become a priest, a social worker, or a school teacher? On the other hand, many are attracted by the special relationship between doctor and patient. This relationship of trust depends on the total honesty of the doctor. It has been said that, "Patients have a uniquely individual relationship with their doctors not encountered in any other profession and anything which undermines patients' confidence in that relationship will ultimately undermine the doctor's ability to carry out his or her work". A journalist writing in the *Sun* wrote cynically, "In truth there is not a single reason to suppose these days that doctors can be trusted any more than you can trust British Gas, a double glazing salesman, or the man in the pub". We disagree—and you would need to disagree too if you were to become a doctor. If it is of any comfort to the *Sun*, a Mori poll in 1999 asked a random selection of the public which professionals could be trusted to tell the truth. The results were: doctors 91%, judges 77%, scientists 63%, business leaders 28%, politicians 23% and journalists 15%.

Professionalism includes the expectation that doctors (and medical students) can be relied on to look after their own health before taking responsibility for the care of others. Doctors who are heavy drinkers or users of prohibited drugs cannot guarantee the necessary clear and consistent judgment, quite apart from the undermining of trust through lawbreaking. Habits start young, and patients have a right to expect high standards of doctors and doctors in training, higher standards than society may demand of others. Those not prepared for such personal discipline have an ethical duty not to choose medicine. It has been said that "Trust is a very fragile thing: it can take years to build up; it takes seconds to destroy". Sir Thomas (later Lord) Bingham, when Master of the Rolls in 1994, expressed the following judgment when rejecting an Appeal by a doctor to the Privy Council against erasure from the medical register at the direction of the Professional Conduct Committee of the GMC. "The reputation of the profession is more important than the fortunes of any individual member. Membership of a profession brings many benefits, but that is part of the price."

The Hippocratic oath is essentially a commitment to absolute honesty, professional integrity, and being a good professional colleague. Many people feel that this spirit is so integral to being a doctor and should be so central to medical education and training that it does not need formal recitation on qualification, especially in the paternalistic phraseology of even modern versions of the Hippocratic oath. On the other hand is there not a place for a formal public declaration by new doctors of their explicit commitment to ethical behaviour? Certainly the graduating medical students at Imperial College in 2001 thought so. They devised their own "affirmation of a new doctor" to etch the association of their new responsibility for the care of patients and promising to act professionally indelibly in their minds—and hearts (see Appendix 1).

The General Medical Council (GMC) is not only responsible for maintaining a register of all doctors licensed to practise medicine in the UK but also for ensuring that doctors are trained to practise and do practise to a high standard. The GMC accepts that the public want to be looked after by doctors who are knowledgeable, skilful, honest, kind and respectful of patients, and who do everything in their power to help them. Above all, that patients want a doctor that they can trust. Explicit duties, responsibilities, values and standards have been clearly set out on behalf of the profession by the GMC in *Good Medical Practice*, which medical students now receive soon after arriving at medical school. Now that contact with patients generally starts early in the course, so does the responsibility of medical students to be professional.

Medicine is an attractive career to good communicators and a difficult one for those who are not. The ability to develop empathy and understanding with all sorts of people in all sorts of situations is an important part of a doctor's art. It is part of medical training, but it helps greatly if it comes naturally in both speaking and writing. A sense of humour and broad interests also assist communication besides helping the doctor to survive as a person. Not all careers in medicine require face to face encounters with patients, but most require good teamwork with other doctors and health workers.

Arrogance, not unknown in the medical profession, hinders both good communication and teamwork. It is not justified: few doctors do things that others with similar training could not do as well—or better. Confidence based on competence and the ability to understand and cope is quite another matter; it is appreciated by patients and colleagues alike. Respect for others and an interest in and concern for their needs is essential. One applicant was getting near the point when she said at interview, "I like people", then paused and continued, "Well, I don't like them all, but I find them interesting". Patients can of course sometimes seem extremely demanding, difficult, unreasonable, and even hostile, particularly when you are exhausted.

5

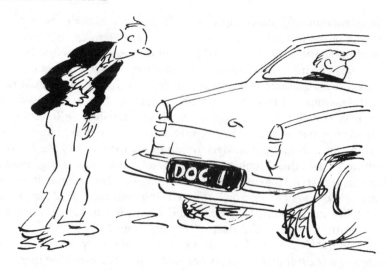

Many people consider medicine because they want to heal. Helping is more common than healing because much human illness is incurable. If curing is your main interest better perhaps become a research pharmacologist developing new drugs. Also, bear in mind that the cost of attempting to cure, whether by drugs or by knife, is sometimes to make matters worse. A doctor must accept and honestly admit uncertainty and fallibility, inescapable parts of many occupations but harder to bear in matters of life and death.

Experience of illness near at hand, in oneself, friends, or family, may reinforce the desire to become a doctor. Having said that, the day to day detail of good care depends more on nurses than doctors and good career opportunities lie there too. In any event, the emotional impact of illness should be taken together with a broader perspective of the realities of the training and the opportunities and obligations of the career. Dr F J Inglefinger, editor of the *New England Journal of Medicine* wrote, when seriously ill himself:

> In medical school, students are told about the perplexity, anxiety and misapprehension that may affect the patient ... and in the clinical years the fortunate and sensitive student may learn much from talking to those assigned to his supervision. But the effects of lectures and conversations are ephemeral and are no substitute for actual experience. One might suggest, of course, that only those who have been hospitalised during their adolescent or adult years be admitted to medical school. Such a practice would not only increase the number of empathic doctors; it would also permit the whole elaborate system of medical school admissions to be jettisoned.

He had his tongue in his cheek, of course, but he also had his heart in his mouth.

Personal experience of the work and life of doctors, first and second hand, preferably in more than one of the different settings of general practice, hospital, or public health, is in any event formative and valuable in getting the feel of whether such work would suit. This can be difficult to arrange while you are still at school, not least because of the confidential nature of the doctor–patient relationship. Observation by a young person who may or may not eventually become a medical student is intrusive and requires great tact from the observer and good will from both doctor and patient. Doctors' children may have an advantage here (the only advantage they do have in the selection process) and could well be expected to know better than others what medical practice is all about. Most applicants have to make do with seeing medicine from another side by helping in hospital, nursing home, or general practitioner's surgery, each situation giving different insights.

And, why not?

Learning medicine involves an education and training longer and more disruptive of personal life than in any other profession. And medicine is moving so fast that doctors can never stop learning. To be trained, it is said, is to have arrived; to be educated is still to be travelling.

Unsocial hours of work are almost inevitable for students and junior doctors and are a continuing obligation in many specialties. If this really is not how you are prepared to spend your life, better not to start than to complain or drop out later. That does not, however, mean that the profession and public has any excuse for failing to press for improvements in working conditions of all doctors, especially for those in training. Exhausted doctors are neither good nor safe, and it becomes difficult for them to profit fully from the lessons of their experience.

What about medicine for a good salary, security, social position, and a job which can in theory be done anywhere? Doctors in the United Kingdom are paid poorly in comparison with other doctors in western Europe, North America, and Australasia, unless they supplement their income with a busy private practice, but, having said that, the pay is not bad. Medicine in the NHS is, above all, still a relatively secure career despite all the recent turmoil, not least because it is now clear that the United Kingdom has for many years trained fewer doctors than it needs and is going to take many years to catch up. Social advancement would be a poor motive, unlikely to achieve its aim. The profession has largely been knocked off its traditional pedestal. Much of the mystery of medicine has been dispelled by good scientific writing and television. Public confidence has been eroded by critical reports of error and incompetence, not to mention a rising tide of litigation against doctors. In the words of Sir Donald Irvine, former president of the GMC: "The public expectation of doctors is changing. Today's patients are better informed. They expect their doctors to behave properly and to perform consistently well, and are less tolerant of poor practice." Such respect that doctors still enjoy has to be continually earned by high standards of professionalism.

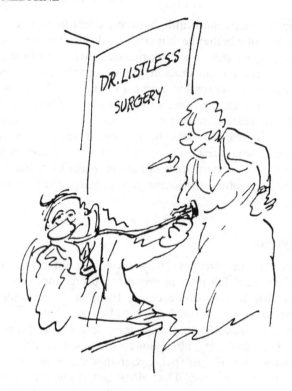

The freedom of doctors to practise in other countries is no longer what it was. Most developed countries have restrictions on doctors trained elsewhere. European Union countries are open to United Kingdom doctors but none is short of doctors, and language barriers have to be overcome. Need and opportunity still exist in developing countries. All in all, there are less demanding ways than medicine of making a good living and having the opportunity to work abroad.

Making your own decision

It would be pompous and old fashioned to insist that all medical students should have a vocation but they do need to be prepared to put themselves out, to *earn* respect, to impose self-discipline, and to take the rough with the smooth in their training and career; they also need to be excited and challenged intellectually and emotionally by some if not all aspects of medicine. And, as much of the decision making in medicine is made on incomplete evidence, they must be able to live with uncertainty. They also need the necessary patience and determination to improve imperfect treatment, increasingly practising "evidence-based" medicine.

It is neither necessary nor normal for individuals to be entirely clear why they want to become a doctor. Those who think they do and also know precisely the sort of doctor they want to be usually change their minds more than once during their training. Whatever your reasons for medicine, the first thing to do is to test your interest as best you can against what the career involves, its demands, its privileges, and its responsibilities. It is not useful to try to decide now what sort of doctor you might want to be, in fact you do not need to decide for at least seven years. But it is wise towards the end of the undergraduate course to examine specialty career options more carefully than most students do now, not least so that enthusiasm about the possibility of a particular specialist career can help motivate you through finals and especially through the somewhat harrowing clinical responsibility of the early postgraduate years.

At the end of the day, your decisions must be your own. If you have questions about course or career, find out who to ask and make your own inquiries; it is your life and your responsibility to make a suitable career choice. Do not let your parents, however willing or however wise, choose your career for you. Beware the fate of Dr Blifil in *Tom Jones* who was described as:

> ... a gentleman who had the misfortune of losing the advantage of great talents by the obstinacy of his father, who would breed him for a profession he disliked ... the doctor had been obliged to study physick [medicine], or rather to say that he had studied it ...

The trust of others, regardless of wealth, poverty, or position, together with the opportunity to understand, explain, and care, if not cure, can bring great fulfilment. So too can the challenge of pushing back the frontiers of medical science and of improving medical practice.

Medicine requires a lively mind, wise judgment, sharp eyes, perceptive hearing, a stout heart, a steady hand, and the ability to learn continuously. It is an ideal career for all rounders and the better rounded you are the wider your career opportunity in medicine as clinician, scientist, teacher, researcher, journalist, or even politician.

Medicine will never be an entirely comfortable or convenient career. It also requires signing up to an ethical code stronger than the law of the land and, even as a student, observing the law—high spirits notwithstanding. Doctors' convictions are never spent. Doctors breaching the law or their ethical code may lose their registration, their licence to practise, and with that their livelihood.

The configuration of an individual's character, aspirations, and abilities have to match the shape of the opportunity, like pegs in holes. Becoming and being a doctor is not by any means everyone's cup of tea. Yet for all its demands, medicine offers a deeply satisfying and rewarding lifetime of service to those prepared to give themselves to it.

REMEMBER

- Becoming a doctor takes five or six years.

- Further postgraduate training takes about as long again.

- There is much to be said both for and against a career in medicine.

- Discover as much as possible about what being a doctor involves before making a decision which will affect the rest of your life.

- Try spending time talking to medical students, hospital doctors, or local GPs.

- The decision for or against applying to medical school should be your own—do not be pressured by school, parents, or friends—it is your life.

2. Opportunity and reality

Statistically, the chances of entry to medical school are pretty good: currently about 12 000 applicants compete for nearly 7000 places, though the current trend of applications is on the increase. Recent moves by the Government to increase the numbers of doctors in the NHS are leading to an increase of available places to 7840 by 2007/08, by building new medical schools and allowing larger numbers of students at existing schools.

In his report, *Learning from Bristol* (2001), Professor Sir Ian Kennedy recommended that:

> Access to medical schools should be widened to include people from diverse academic and socio-economic backgrounds. Those with qualifications in other areas of healthcare and those with educational background in subjects other than science, who have the ability and wish to, should have greater opportunities than is presently the case, to enter medical school.

In fact, most medical schools will consider applicants without a strong science background, especially for some graduate entry courses.

Most applicants come from professional or clerical backgrounds. Many others still see medicine as a closed shop in which, if you do not have such a background, you stand little chance of either entry or success. Research has shown that once academic ability has been discounted neither social class, age, medical relatives, nor type of secondary school affect chances of entry to medical school. But examination results depend partly on educational opportunity at school, not to mention encouragement to study at home. Some medical schools try to make some allowance for this.

The fact of the matter is that many people simply do not believe they have a real opportunity to become a doctor. Many who might well make excellent doctors and would broaden the perspectives and insights of the medical profession as a whole simply do not apply. If they do not apply, they cannot be considered.

Academic achievement is the most important determinant of success in selection. Some medical schools make their final selection on grades alone; most also take account of attitudes, personality, and broader achievements, qualities which being difficult to measure require judgment to assess and therefore cannot be proved to be absolutely fair. Nevertheless, an immense amount of effort is put into making selection as fair as possible.

The long course of study, diminishing educational grants, mounting student debts, and course fees also tend to deter those without financial backing. It is extremely difficult to work one's way through medical school. Spare time jobs are difficult to find, and the course leaves little time for them, especially in the later years with on call duties in hospital. The fact that the job is secure at the end of the road and is sufficiently well paid for debts to be repaid seems just too far away to be any consolation.

Opportunities for women

Universities across the world were slow to give women equal opportunity to higher education, and medicine was perhaps the slowest professional course of all. Several United Kingdom medical schools first admitted women as students only 50 years ago (except during the world wars when they were unable to fill all their places with men).

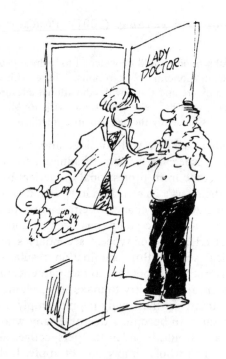

Women now have equal opportunity to enter medicine. In 1991, for the first time, more women than men were admitted to medical school in the United Kingdom, and the following year, for the first time women predominated among both applicants and entrants. This trend continues, and in 2001 the proportions of women and men in both applications and entrants was about 58% women and 42% men. Such is the turn around of the imbalance of men and women students that some admissions tutors are asking if the time has come to consider ways of encouraging male applicants, although there is as yet no talk of quotas or positive action for men!

Although it can still be argued that the medical profession as a whole is still male dominated, there is no doubt that as the trend towards more women students continues, this is being slowly but surely broken down by sheer force of the numbers of women doctors. Some specialties remain more challenging for women to succeed in than others, but some fields are naturally finding the majority of their new recruits are women.

In the past, careers advisers, parents, and applicants were understandably aware of the potential personal conflicts ahead between career and family at a time when, even more than today, women were left holding the baby while the man got on with his career. Times have changed, and society's attitudes to parenting are changing all the time. Also the conflict between career and personal interests is not confined to women and to bringing up a family. Some argue positively for medicine as being better placed than many other careers for resolving this conflict, as Dr Susan Andrew has done:

> Medicine is a most suitable career for intelligent, educated women who aspire to married life, because it carries far more opportunities for flexible working than other professions ... My message is: remember, women have struggled for centuries to have lives of their own and to be defined in terms of their own achievements, not someone else's.

Ethnic minorities

Medicine, science, and engineering are all disproportionately popular university courses with home students from ethnic minorities, especially those of Indian or south east Asian origin. More than a quarter of home applicants to medical school are drawn from ethnic minorities, although they comprise less than one tenth of the United Kingdom population. Afro-Caribbeans are an exception, reflecting their current general academic underachievement, a cause of national concern; medical schools are keen to encourage them to apply.

Concern has also been expressed that applicants from ethnic minorities with equivalent academic grades were found a few years ago to be less likely to be shortlisted for interview; once interviewed, however, they were as likely to receive an offer as anyone else. The difference was small, less than the disadvantage of applying towards the end of the application period, but it still existed in a survey in 1998. One reason may be that these applicants have had less opportunity and encouragement to develop leadership skills, to pursue wider interests, and to participate in community service, all important dimensions at shortlisting in most medical schools. Prejudice may also have been a factor because a similar disadvantage has been found in shortlisting for junior hospital posts. A study a few years ago showed that when identical CVs were submitted under different names, those bearing a European name were more likely to be shortlisted than others for senior house officer posts. Since 1998 stringent steps have been taken in all medical schools to ensure equal opportunities, and no recent evidence has caused concern.

A small but significant minority of Indian or Asian women students experience family pressures which undermine their ability to cope happily or effectively with their academic work. Parents and grandparents may curtail freedom, command frequent presence (a demand not limited to the women students or indeed to Asian families), and occasionally impose arranged marriages. Deans are familiar with situations in which they have to send down students for academic failure due to such pressures. Parents must better understand that until the pressures that are preventing their child from working effectively are removed—by giving them more personal and intellectual liberty—they have no prospect of being readmitted to a medical course.

Of course, families of any section of society can place pressures on a student—such as a young student who has to care for younger siblings or an elderly relative. While these pressures are understandable, and often, inadvertent, can it ever be acceptable to undermine a young person's chances in life, however difficult the family circumstances?

Mature students

Age is statistically no disadvantage in application to medical school, but that may well be because few mature students have the necessary academic and financial credentials to apply. Most medical schools restrict consideration to those aged under 30 or discourage those older than that, even if not actually excluding them from open competition with equally bright younger applicants, perhaps as committed (even if less experienced) and with potentially an extra decade of service to offer as a doctor. Less than 1% of entrants to medical school are over 30 when they start, only 3% are between 25 and 30, and 6% between 21 and 24. Deans have a difficult balancing act to perform. Some years ago as a way of challenging a mature applicant at interview to make her case, I said, "If we offer you a place the phone will ring and the prime minister will ask how we can possibly justify national investment in you rather than in a younger person", at which moment the telephone on my desk rang. It was not the prime minister, and the applicant won her place.

Most medical schools welcome the contribution mature students make to the stability and responsibility of their year group and more widely within the medical school as a result of their greater experience, achievement, and compassion. Maturity helps in communicating and empathising with patients, to the extent that many deans would prefer to take all their students over the age of 21.

Good organisation, a sufficient income, and an understanding partner with a flexible job (if any partner at all) are the foundations of successful medical study by mature students with family responsibilities. The early years of the course are no more difficult for medicine than other degree courses, except in that the intensity of lectures and practical work is greater than in most other subjects. Efficient use of time during the day and a regular hour or two of study most evenings (with more before examinations) should suffice. Some students manage to support themselves for a year or two by evening and weekend jobs. It is not easy and becomes more or less impossible during the later years, when the working year is 48 weeks. Most clinical assignments require one night or weekend in hospital every week or two. Two or three "residences"—for example, in obstetrics or paediatrics—may require living in a distant hospital for a week or two at a time, learning as one of the medical team by day and sometimes at night. An increasing number of schools are farming out their students to district hospitals—often some miles from the university town—for much longer periods of time than before. If this is likely to cause major problems with some students it is worth checking this out before you choose where to apply. The working day at that stage is long, starting at 8.00 am and finishing about 5.00 pm or later, with most weekends free. The elective period of two or three months is often spent abroad but may be spent close to home and does not necessarily entail night or weekend duty. Finally, several weeks as a shadow house officer involves residence in hospital at the end of the course.

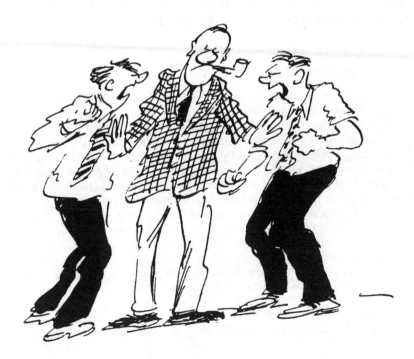

Some mature students manage magnificently. One who started just over the age of 30 and had two children aged between 5 and 10 and a husband willing and able to adjust his working hours to hers had studied for A levels when she was a busy mother. Her further education college described her as the most academically and personally outstanding student that they could remember; she won several prizes on her way through medical school and qualified without difficulty. Another of similar age with four children and separated from her husband, coped with such amazing energy and effectiveness, despite considerable financial hardship (and the help of a succession of competent and reliable au pairs) that she left everyone breathless. Exceptional these two may be, but it can be done, requiring as Susan Spindler commented in her book, *Doctors To Be*, "an unerring sense of priorities in her life, tremendous stamina and the capacity to concentrate briefly but hard".

Mature students are at a substantial financial disadvantage if they have already had a student loan for higher education. Even if eligible for bursaries or additional loans, those who have already achieved financial independence find their reduced circumstances tough.

Finance is only one of the problems facing mature students: to revert from being an independent individual to becoming one of a bunch of recent school leavers can be both hard and tiresome, although most mature students in medicine seem to cope with this transition remarkably well. Shorter courses (four years) for some graduates have now been introduced at several universities, with students supported for the last three years by NHS bursaries (see page 39). Better let a mature student, an Oxford graduate in psychology, give her own impressions:

The mature student's tale

I have always felt that the term "mature student" is vaguely uncomplimentary— almost synonymous with "fuddy old fart" or "bearded hippy". Personally I have never considered myself particularly "mature" in comparison with my year group, while others merely describe themselves as being slightly less immature. Some of us have had previous jobs ranging from city slicker to nurse or army officer, while others may have come straight from a previous degree or are supporting a family. Whatever the difference in background one common factor unites us all, we are convinced that medicine is now the career for us. Deciding this a little later than most brings its own particular problems.

To start with, the interview tends to be rather different to that of a school leaver. There are usually only three questions that the panel really want answering. Firstly, why did you decide to study medicine now? Is it a realistic decision, or just a diversion from a midlife crisis, do you know what the job actually entails, and how can you assure them you will not change your mind again? Secondly, "How do you think you will cope being *so* much older than everybody else", which I found rather patronising, but it is wise to have thought of a suitable response. Thirdly—and most importantly—how will you finance yourself? No medical school wants to give a place to someone who will subsequently drop out due to financial pressure.

Most mature medical students undoubtedly find that the financial burden poses the biggest problem. While it is possible to finance yourself through scholarships, charities, loans, and overdrafts, this takes a lot of time and organisation. Most medical schools still want a financial guarantor in addition. Many students get a part time job to ease the pressure but during a heavily timetabled and examined medical course this can prove difficult. Progression through to the clinical years brings even fewer opportunities for work with unpredictable hours and scarce holidays. It is worth investigating which medical schools and universities are more accepting of mature students, and which have funds to help financially. Aside from the obvious practical problems of having little money, coping with the financial divide between yourself and old friends now earning can take some getting used to.

Once the financial issues have been hurdled, other worries surface. Fitting in with school leavers may initially be viewed as a problem, but if you can survive Freshers' Week I can assure you it does get easier. Progressing through the course the proportion of shared experience increases and the initial age and experience gap no longer poses such a problem. One particular advantage of the length of the medical course is that those in the final year may be of a similar age to those entering as mature students, and due to the wide range of clubs and societies offered by most universities there is ample opportunity to meet people of all ages.

One advantage of being that little bit older is that it is much easier not to feel you have to succumb to the peer group pressure so often prevalent in the medical school environment. When faced with the tempting offer to stand naked on a table and down a yard of ale, the excuse "I've got to get home to the wife and kids" will usually suffice.

The attitude of some medical students to those older than themselves can occasionally be somewhat disconcerting. A first year student was recently heard to comment to a mature student in her year, "Isn't it funny, you are in our year, but when we come back for reunions, you will probably be dead."

A variety of roles may be created by your new peer group for you to fit in to. These can range from being initially seen as the "old freak" or "year swot" to pseudo parent or agony aunt. These roles do tend to diminish over time, and most mature students are viewed as an asset as they bring in a different range of knowledge and experience. The importance of maintaining old friendships and having an outlet away from medicine, however, cannot be overemphasised.

"Will I be able to cope with the work?" can obviously be a further worry. A levels may seem a dim and distant memory, and the type of work or learning most mature students have been previously doing is a far cry from the vast amounts of memorising required by the medical course. There is no doubt about it—studying medicine is a lot of work, with regular exams and a full timetable. Most mature students do seem to have developed a better notion of time management and efficient learning, however, and this, coupled with a strong motivation to complete the course, can alleviate some of the work pressure.

Being a clinical student learning on the wards brings its own particular problems. The transition from having a respected job or being an instrumental part of a team to having no exact role perhaps presents more difficulties to a mature student than to others. The unpleasant "teaching by humiliation" method employed by some doctors may be particularly trying to mature students, especially when (as has been known to happen) the person being so patronising was in your little sister's year at school. Being at the very bottom of such an entrenched hierarchy can be wearing and frustrating. Overall, however, most doctors involved in teaching are extremely supportive of mature students, and a proportion feel all medical students should gain outside experience before embarking on a medical career.

Progressing through the training the clinical aspects of the course become more important and, for the majority of students, more enjoyable. Mature students tend to find this especially true and are often in a position of strength, being more confident and relaxed in their interactions with patients, bringing skills and experience from previous careers. Personally I have found this one of the greatest assets of being a mature student, finding emotional or difficult situations easier to cope with than if I had come straight into medicine from school.

The downside can be that fellow students and doctors can have a higher expectation of your abilities and knowledge. While this may be true in some aspects of communication, the learning curve for practical skills is just the same as for others. Being a few years older does not necessarily mean you are an instant pro at inserting a catheter.

Once you have realistically decided that medicine is the career for you, possibly sat required A levels, got through the interview, and faced up to the prospect of at least five years' financial hardship, is it all worth it?

Being a mature student it is all the more important to make sure that the decision to study medicine is not viewed idealistically. There are some doctors who deeply regret the decision to go into the profession. One doctor, who was a mature student, replied when asked, "It was the worst decision I ever made. I'm permanently tired and just don't have the time I would like for myself or family anymore."

Older students obviously often have different commitments and priorities which their younger colleagues are yet to experience, such as children or a mortgage. While life through medical school can be hard, with academic stress and financial worry, difficulties do not end with qualification. Becoming a doctor not only brings new opportunities but also a different way of life. The line between work and personal life can become increasingly blurred. Despite a more enlightened approach to junior doctors' hours, the time commitment is still immense. The work ethic is unlike that of any other career. This means that inevitable sacrifices have to be made in one's personal life, and consideration as to how this will affect present or future partners and children is important.

Having stated many of the difficulties, the advantages of being a mature student are considerable. Medicine, perhaps more than any other profession, requires a maturity of insight, both personally and in dealing with patients; many situations are emotionally demanding and stressful; coping with added academic pressure can be tiring and demoralising. A more mature approach together with a greater certainty in your career choice is a definite asset.

Maintaining friendships outside medicine means that when it all gets a bit too much you can escape, and being offered a second chance at being a student can mean you make far more of the opportunities offered to you than when you first left school. Overall I have found medicine to be fascinating and enjoyable. The career choices available once you are in the profession are extremely varied so finding your niche should be possible. The combination of human contact with academic interest is unlike that of any other career, and the unique privilege of being so intimately involved in people's lives never fails to be exciting or interesting. It *is* possible and personally I feel it *is* worth it ... (but ask me again when I'm a junior doctor).

SE

Overseas applicants

Overseas students are in a competition of their own for reserved places, amounting to 7·5% of the total national intake of medical students. About 1500 overseas students compete for about 330 places, giving them about the same chance of a place as home students. The recent increases in medical schools' places, however, were a response to staffing problems in the NHS, and so none of the new medical schools are able at present to admit overseas students; this is currently under review. Students from the European Union count as home students. Overseas students are liable for full fees, amounting to a total of about £65 000 over five years. They will also need about £50 000 for their living expenses. It is no longer possible for someone from overseas to be classified as a home student by purchasing secondary education at a British school, by nominating a "guardian" with a United Kingdom address, or by buying a United Kingdom residence. Nor are British expatriates working permanently abroad normally eligible for home fee status.

Local education authorities (LEA) are responsible for finally determining fee status; the guidelines state that students are able to pay fees at the home rate only if they have been "ordinarily resident" in the United Kingdom or in a member state of the European Union in the previous three years and have not been resident during any part of that period wholly or mainly for the purpose of receiving full time education. Exception is made for nationals or their children who have not been ordinarily resident during that period because of temporary employment abroad. Officially recognised refugees and people granted asylum or exceptional leave to remain in the United Kingdom are also treated as exceptions.

Overseas students are entitled to stay for four years and sometimes longer after graduation to undertake their specialist postgraduate medical education in the United Kingdom, in which capacity they make a welcome contribution as junior doctors.

Equal opportunities, equal difficulties?

Opportunity to enter medicine has, as far as can be judged, become equal for those realistic about their qualifications. But everyone considering becoming a doctor must look behind and beyond medical school to the reality of whether a career in medicine is for them a pathway to fulfilment or to frustration. The tension between the relative freedom of many careers and the ties of medicine face men and women alike. But medicine is a tougher career for many women than for most men. A few years ago we received a letter from three students from St George's Hospital Medical School in London, indignant about the suggestion that the position of women requires special consideration: "For a start, let's bury the idea that male and female students have different aspirations—we all wish to end up well rounded human beings..." Sure, but it is not necessary to become a doctor to do that, although medical education will have failed in part of its purpose if all doctors are not "well rounded" individuals.

The difficulties particularly facing women doctors are both subtle and unsubtle. The obvious are the dual responsibilities of family and career, which most women do not wish to know about, consider, or even recognise when they are medical students but which they begin to come to terms with once the all consuming task of qualifying as a doctor has been achieved. Opportunities for part time training and employment in many specialties are limited. Career dice are loaded against those who patiently plod through long years of part time training. Progress towards a training and a career structure which would fully harness skills of (in future) at least half the medical workforce is slow. The personal and national cost of failure to use the skills of women doctors fully would be immense.

The potential disadvantages for women in postgraduate training can be and often are overcome supremely well with good family support. Recent changes in taxation allowances also mean better financial support for working families through tax relief on childcare. Some specialties—such as general practice, pathology, radiology, anaesthetics, and public health—can readily be made flexible and compatible with other responsibilities.

The more subtle difficulties facing women include the feeling that more is demanded of them as doctors because they are women. Not all women agree but a woman doctor, Fran Reichenberg, wrote that:

> Both patients and staff expect far more of female doctors. These expectations arise from traditional female roles in society of mother, carer, soother of the distressed ...

She also believed that male doctors may get special treatment from the team:

> The perks of the male house officer who shows a clear interest in the female staff include his ivs being drawn up and done, his results filed for him, his blood forms filled out. Many telephone calls chasing results being done for

him. ... These differences amount to many extra hours' work a week for the female house officer and exacerbate her fatigue and low morale.

In our experience, special treatment can work both ways.

Women compete very effectively but sometimes against the odds. The unsaid concern about the organisational and financial impact of maternity leave seems to confer no overall disadvantage. Women may, however, suffer disproportionately from the innate conservatism of consultant appointments committees. Most members of appointments committees and most remaining consultants in post are for historical reasons men. Having more women on appointments committees is not necessarily the answer: on one occasion the strongest opposition to taking gender into account in appointing to an obstetric team serving an ethnic population with substantial preferences for women doctors came from the only woman on the committee.

Many women still feel at a disadvantage, as Dr Anne Nicol, a consultant pathologist, explained:

> Unless we remove the glass ceiling, many top candidates for consultant posts will fail to reach the top. Let's face it, jobs go to the applicant wanted by the consultants in post ... [who] still see the ideal colleague as someone much like themselves ... you can almost hear them say "one has to be able to get on with him—he has to be on your wave length" ... tribalism among male consultants is strong, pressure to be one of the herd intense; Tory voting, middle class, privately educated, golf playing white males are the tribal group most likely to succeed ...

> The common perception is that women don't fit in, are difficult to work with and can never be one of the tribe. A woman making a vocal stance on a topic will find it is not long before someone comments on her hormonal balance or time of month ...

> We can ensure that more women at least get their noses pressed against the glass ceiling by creating more family friendly training packages, part time posts and job shares.

Each aspiring entrant to medicine must come to terms with the length and the nature of the training, the demands of the career, and the reality of his or her own personality and ability. Add to this a strategic view of the opportunity—open and equal on merit at the beginning, convoluted later for several reasons, but destined to become more equal. Finally, the professional responsibility of putting patients first is inescapable, often uncomfortable, but fulfilling.

REMEMBER

- Anyone with ability and aptitude stands a chance of admission to medical school; background does not matter.

- Once academic achievement has been taken into account, social class, age, having parents who are doctors, or the type of school you attended will not affect your chances of admission.

- Being a woman gives a slight but statistically significant increase in your chances.

- Mature students are welcomed by most medical schools but they often have to overcome both financial and personal difficulties.

- Shorter courses (usually four years) are now available at an increasing number of schools for graduates in science or health related subjects.

- Students with children will need good home support.

- About 7·5% of places at UK medical schools are reserved for overseas students, their chance of admission is similar to home students.

3. Requirements for entry

Entry to medical school is academically the most competitive moment in the student's life. However, becoming a doctor requires many more qualities than brain power, including compassion, endurance, determination, communication skills, enthusiasm, intellectual curiosity, balance, adaptability, integrity and a sense of humour. All these are highly desirable attributes but not absolute "requirements" for entry to medicine: few have them all but a remarkable number of applicants have many.

Academic ability is an essential requirement for entry, and the ability to pass examinations remains important throughout the course and the subsequent years of postgraduate training. Less competitive than A levels, but no less intense, were the traditional end of first and second year examinations on the sciences underpinning medicine. New curriculums that emphasise understanding and integration of knowledge rather than "facts" are tested more by continuous assessment, a less destructive process than a series of annual crises but not without a constantly recurring academic tension. Professionally, the hardest exams are those for the higher specialist diplomas of fellowship or membership of the medical Royal Colleges, requiring a broad and solid grasp of the clinical skills, knowledge, and, to an increasing extent, the attitudes appropriate to a specialist. "Finals"—the examinations for the Bachelor of Medicine and Surgery degree, the degree which acts as the basis for a provisional licence to practise as a doctor, are largely a matter of hard slog, particularly in the later years. They used to be taken as a big bang at the end of the course but are now broken up at most universities over a period of about 18 months.

Broader requirements

Although all doctors need to be bright (not less perhaps than what it takes to get three B grades at A level at first attempt), medicine needs a great deal more than academic ability. With the headlong advance of science and technology, it is no longer true to say that "the A level requirements select people too academic for a career which needs compassion, endurance, and a damn good memory rather than brains", but those qualities certainly are still needed. Compassion is easier to detect in someone who has already shown practical concern for others, perhaps in voluntary, social, or medically related work (such as helping with remedial teaching of younger and less able pupils at school or working in a local hospital or nursing home on one's own initiative rather than simply as a requirement for voluntary work at school). It impresses most admissions tutors to see applicants whom, in their UCAS form personal statements, can show a longer commitment to such work than the odd day here or there, or perhaps a week of work experience organised by school, as most applicants will have done this. This element of past experience often forms popular subject matter for any interview panel, so make sure you have something interesting to say about it and how it has informed your decision to study medicine. The ability to communicate well, to work in a team with a confident but not arrogant manner, and to be prepared as need arises to lead and take responsibility is important too. A sense of humour sprinkles oil on the wheels of communication.

Endurance, determination, and perseverance are part of the same package. They feed on dual enthusiasm for science and for the healing art

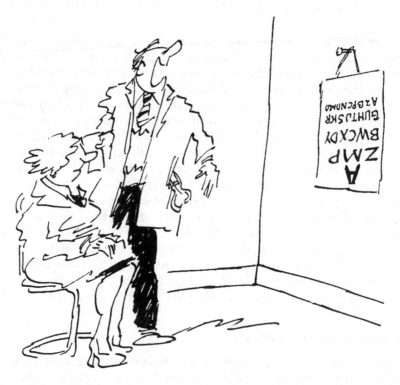

of medicine. They are inspired by curiosity and enriched by sparks of initiative and originality. Lord Moran (Dean of St Mary's and Winston Churchill's doctor) once said, "The student who is not curious is surely no student at all; he is already old, and his thoughts are borrowed thoughts."

Becoming a doctor is not as formidable as it sounds, given good friends, teachers, and opportunities to learn, but it requires solid organisation of time and life and being self propelled. Desirable characteristics for medicine do not end here. Balance is needed, balance which comes from an intellectual and personal life broader and deeper than academic success alone. Professor David Greenfield, first Dean of the University of Nottingham Medical School, referred to "balance of scientific and clinical excellence, humanitarian and compassionate concern ... balance of service and learning, balance of current competence and future adaptability". Other interests—literary, musical, artistic, and sporting—encourage achievement, provide recreation, and demand application, enthusiasm, and ability. They can become great stabilisers and good points of communication with both colleagues and patients. For a female accident and emergency consultant to also be the medical officer for a well known football club (not that she is a great player) is good for her and for her hospital.

Then there is the invaluable down to earth ability to organise and to cope; a capable pair of hands and a reassuring attitude of "leave it to me and I'll sort it out", taking huge weights off shoulders and loads off minds. Sir George Pickering, onetime Regius Professor of Medicine at Oxford, wrote, "Medicine is in some ways the most personal and responsible profession: the patient entrusts his life and wellbeing to his doctor. Thus, the character and personality of the doctor, his sympathy and understanding, his sense of responsibility, his selflessness are as important as his scientific and technical knowledge." He also pointed out that a doctor neither needs to nor should try to sort out every problem him or herself: "the best doctors know to whom to turn for help".

Many medical schools, when asked which qualities they regarded as most important in applicants to medicine, highlighted the desirability of a realistic understanding of what is demanded in the study of medicine and in the subsequent career. Without this embryo insight many years of unhappiness may lie ahead, however bright and however gifted the student. Failure to understand the demands of the job and the limitations of the art may explain why some doctors drop out of medicine.

Applicants from medical backgrounds have an advantage in this respect. They have seen the effects of the career on their parents and families and have had the opportunity to explore what their parent or parents do; they also have relatively easy access to observing other medical specialties. All the more regrettable if they have not taken this opportunity to find out what it's all about. For others, it is much more difficult. Most TV medical programmes glamorise and trivialise and give little insight into the everyday undramatic life of a doctor. The BBC TV series *Doctors To Be* and *Doctors At Large*, following students through their years at St Mary's, and now for ten years into their careers, are an exception and offer useful insights, even if the structure of the course itself has now changed. The rather embattled and disillusioned group of new doctors at the end of the series has now been balanced by glimpses of where they are now, ten years on, and reveals that they feel that it has all been worth while. Because this is one of the most fundamental aspects of making an informed personal decision *Learning Medicine* puts less emphasis on the years in medical school and more on where they lead.

Personal health requirements and disability

A doctor's overriding responsibility is the safety and well-being of patients. As such all applicants to medical school must have the potential to function as a fully competent doctor and fulfil the rigorous demands of professional fitness to practice as stated by the General Medical Council. All applicants must therefore disclose any disabilities or medical conditions on the application form as they may affect the ability to practise medicine. This may be by placing patients at risk of infection, being unable to perform necessary medical procedures, or by impairing your judgment. Similarly applicants must also complete a declaration that they have no criminal convictions or pending prosecutions, in line with national policies for staff working in sensitive roles. In most circumstances a declaration does not automatically disqualify an applicant but will allow the case to be decided on its own merits.

The UK Department of Health has requirements for specific conditions, which means that a student cannot be admitted with active tuberculosis or if infectious with hepatitis B, until they can be proven to be no longer infectious. In the case of hepatitis B, all prospective students must show proof of adequate immunisation before commencing the course. You will be asked for documentary proof when you arrive at medical school. Your own GP can usually arrange for hepatitis B immunisation to be carried out. The course and testing for a satisfactory response can take up to nine months, so you should discuss this with your GP at the earliest opportunity. If there is a failure to respond to the immunisation a student will be expected to prove that they are not infectious. In these rare circumstances, or where a student tests positive for any of the hepatitis B antigens, they should discuss this with their GP and the admissions tutor of their preferred school, as soon as possible.

There is no clear national policy as yet about candidates who are known to be hepatitis C positive. However, this must be declared on the UCAS form, and individual schools will advise in this rare instance. In any event, failure to disclose any condition that puts patients at risk will result in immediate dismissal from medical school.

All students are advised to be immunised against meningococcal meningitis before starting at university.

Any disability should also be disclosed and will be dealt with by the schools on a case by case basis. Dyslexia should also be disclosed on the UCAS form and this will need to be supported by a formal statement from a suitably qualified psychologist. Most medical schools will advise relevant departments of the assistance which may be necessary for students with dyslexia and will make some time allowances in written examinations, but no concessions are made in clinical examinations.

Taking illegal drugs or abusing alcohol are also inconsistent with a doctor's professional responsibilities, both on patient safety grounds and the need for personal integrity. Students who ignore their responsibilities to be utterly dependable in this regard put their place in medical school in severe jeopardy.

Academic requirements

Although academic achievement is only the qualifying standard for entering the real field of selection, like the Olympic qualifying standard is to selection for the national team, it is overwhelmingly the strongest element in selection. Unlike all the other desirable attributes of personality, attitude, and interest examination results look deceptively objective. Relatively objective they may be but they are still poor indicators of the potential to become "a good doctor"—a product difficult to define, not least because medicine is such a wide career that there may be many different sorts of good doctors—but they all need the appropriate knowledge, skills, and attitudes for effective medical practice and the ability to use them competently.

Examination results at the age of 18 do not predict late developers nor do they take account of differences in educational opportunity at school nor of support for study at home. Results may also be upset by ill health on the day; even minor illness or discomfort crucially timed may take the gloss off the performance, a gloss which may make all the difference between a place at medical school and no place at all. Having said that, however, those who fail during the medical course are generally those with the poorest A level results, and those who do best, especially in the early years with their greater scientific content, are generally those with the highest. But there are outstanding exceptions.

All medical schools set a minimum standard of at least ABB at A level (Table 3.1). The actual achievement of entrants is very similar at all universities whatever their target requirements, except Oxford and Cambridge, where they are higher. Medical schools which set marginally lower grades leave themselves the flexibility to make allowances for special situations and to give due weight to outstanding non-academic attributes. Most successful applicants to medical schools setting a lower minimum substantially exceed their requirements. It is vital to realise that good grades do not guarantee a place: far more applicants achieve the necessary grades than can be given a place.

Chemistry or physical science is required by all universities for medicine. They prefer this at A level, but practically all of the medical schools in the United Kingdom are prepared to accept AS chemistry in place of A level. Most are prepared to accept a combination of AS levels in place of another science or maths A level. In practice AS levels are normally offered in addition to three A levels and not in substitution for one. The detailed requirements can be found in the UCAS *Students Guide to Entry to Medicine* and should if in doubt be double checked with the medical school in question. Many universities prefer two other science subjects at A level,

27

Table 3.1—Typical grades required at first attempt for entry to medicine excluding premedical, 1st MB, courses

Medical school	Grades
Birmingham	AAB
Brighton & Sussex *minus*	ABB
Bristol −5 yrs. including BSc (European) *&*	AAB
Cambridge • 5yrs. including BA in MedSci	AAA
East Anglia	AAB
Hull–York	ABB
Leeds	AAB
Leicester–Warwick	AAB
Liverpool	ABB
Imperial College, London −6yrs. including BSc	ABB
King's College, London (Guys, King's, St Thomas')− 5yrs. minus BSc	ABB
Queen Mary's, London (Bart's & Royal London)	ABB
St George's London	ABB
University College, London (Royal Free & University College)− 6yrs +BSc	ABB
Manchester − 5 yr. minus BSc (European)	AAB
Newcastle	AAB
Nottingham −5 yrs. including BSc	AAB
Oxford − 5 yrs. + BA in Physiology	AAA
Peninsula	AAB
Sheffield	ABB
Southampton	AAB
Aberdeen	ABB
Dundee	ABB
Edinburgh	AAB
Glasgow	AAB
St Andrew's	ABB
University of Wales College of Medicine, Cardiff	AAB
Queen's University, Belfast	AAB

All medical schools are prepared to accept one and sometimes more than one non-science or maths A level.

See medical school prospectuses or websites for more details if non A level entrance qualifications will be offered.

taken from the group of physics (unless physical science is offered), biology, and mathematics, but all are prepared to accept a good grade in an arts subject in place of one, or in some medical schools, two science subjects. Some medical schools do not accept maths and higher maths together as two of the required three A level subjects. General studies A level is generally not acceptable as one of the subjects.

No particular non-science subjects are favoured but knowledge based rather than practical skills based subjects are generally preferred. It may be difficult to compare grades in arts and science subjects, so a higher target may be set for an arts subject for entry to medicine. Several universities express a preference for biology over physics or maths. Chemistry and biology are the foundations of medical science, especially if the mathematical aspects of those subjects are included. But however useful it is to be numerate in medicine, especially in research, students without a good knowledge of biology find themselves handicapped at least in the first year of the course by their lack of understanding of cell and organ function and its terminology. They also generally have greater difficulty in expressing themselves in writing, especially if their first language is not English. Failure in the first two years of the medical course is more common in those who did not take biology at A level. All universities require good grades in science and mathematics at GCSE level if not offered at A level, together with English language.

The relative popularity with applicants of mathematics over biology does not indicate changed perception of the value of mathematics for medicine but reflects the general usefulness of maths for entry to alternative science courses. It may also be because good mathematicians (or average mathematicians with good teachers) can expect higher grades in mathematics than in the more descriptive subject of biology. A few applicants gain excellent grades at A level in four subjects—for example, chemistry, physics, biology, and mathematics or the less appropriate combination for medicine of chemistry, physics or biology, mathematics, and higher mathematics. It is a better strategy for admission to achieve three good grades than four indifferent ones.

Scottish Highers are the usual entry qualification offered by Scottish applicants, most of whom apply to study at Scottish medical schools. Scottish qualifications are accepted by medical schools in England, Wales, and Northern Ireland. Most have hitherto required a good pass in the certificate of sixth year studies (CSYS), but with the introduction of new Scottish Highers and Advanced Highers the CSYS has disappeared. The Scottish academic tests are accompanied by formal testing of core study skills needed for understanding a university course: personal effectiveness and problem solving, communication, numeracy, and information technology.

Both the International Baccalaureate and the European Baccalaureate are acceptable entry qualifications at United Kingdom medical schools but only a handful of entrants come by that route. Requirements vary at different schools and can be found in the UCAS publication. Even fewer students enter medicine with BTEC/SCOT BTEC National Diploma Certificate but it is a possible route of entry. The Advanced General National Vocational Qualification (GNVQ) or General Scottish Vocational Qualification (GSVQ) are not generally accepted, although some universities are prepared to consider it on an individual basis. It is likely that a distinction would be required, along with a high grade in GCE A level, probably in chemistry. Over half the medical schools in the UK will accept as an entry qualification the Access to Medicine Certificate from the College of West Anglia in King's Lynn (www.col-westanglia.ac.uk). This is a one year full time course in physics, chemistry, and biology designed for potential applicants to medical schools with good academic backgrounds or professional qualifications, such as in nursing.

Graduate students

Most medical schools will accept applications from graduates for the conventional course. A first or upper second class honours degree is usually required, most commonly in a science or health related subject. Unless their degree includes chemistry or biochemistry, an A level in chemistry is usually required in addition. It may be acceptable for a graduate to sit the GAMSAT (Graduate Australian Medical School Admissions Test), a scientific aptitude test which is usually held once a year, for example at St George's Hospital Medical School. A good score in this, in addition to their degree and personal characteristics may be acceptable. Students wishing to pursue this method of entry are best advised to contact their preferred schools early to discuss this option. In addition a growing number of medical schools have started—or are planning to introduce—shortened (four year) medical courses for some graduates (see page 40). These courses generally condense the early years and basic science component of the course. Similarly those schools with six year courses that include an intercalated BSc or equivalent, such as Oxford, Imperial College, and Royal Free and University College Medical School are introducing shorter (five year) courses if you already have a similar degree. If the degree includes chemistry or biochemistry, it may be accepted in lieu of A level chemistry, otherwise this is likely to be required in addition. Graduate entrants are not normally exempted from any parts of the medical course at most medical schools but they are in some.

How about resits?

What about those who take longer before a first attempt or retake examinations after further study, having failed to achieve their grade target at first attempt? Clearly, there are perfectly understandable reasons for poor performance at first attempt, such as illness, bereavement, and multiple change of school, which most medical schools are prepared to take into account, at least if they had judged the candidate worthy of an offer in the first place. Medical schools which did not give an offer first time round are unlikely to make an offer at second attempt. Apart from these exceptions, most medical schools are not normally prepared to consider applicants who failed to obtain high grades at first attempt.

Three points might be made about applicants who, for no good reason, perform below target at first attempt. Firstly, a modest polishing of grades confers little additional useful knowledge and gives no promise of improved potential for further development, especially when only one or two subjects are retaken. The less there is to do the better it should be done, and the medical course itself requires the ability to keep several subjects on the boil simultaneously. On the other hand, a dramatic improvement (unless achieved by highly professional cramming) may indicate late development or reveal desirable and necessary qualities of determination and application. Secondly, age should be taken into account. The usual age for taking A level is 18, and some much younger applicants may simply have been taken through school too fast. Thirdly, those unlikely to achieve ABB at GCE A level (or equivalent) at first attempt are probably unwise to be thinking of medicine, unless their non-academic credentials are very strong indeed. Even then, it is likely to be an uphill battle. Read the prospectus carefully between the lines to try to discover those medical schools most likely to give weight to broader achievements.

Survival ability

So much for what we think medical schools are, or should be, looking for. But what qualities are needed for survival? We asked Susan Spindler, producer of *Doctors To Be*, what in her opinion, based on several years in medical school and hospital making the TV series, makes a good medical student. This is what she said:

Medical school is very hard work and great fun. There will be a vast array of things to do in your free time coupled with a syllabus that could have you working day and night for years. You need to be the sort of person who can keep both opportunities and work requirements in perspective. There is a lot of drinking and a lot of sport. In many universities the burden of the curriculum and the emotional pressure of the course means that medics tend to stick together and intense, but rather narrow, friendships can result. Try to make and maintain friendships with non-medics. Many medical schools aim to select gregarious, confident characters who have experience of facing and overcoming challenges and leading others. It certainly helps if you fit this mould—but there are many successful exceptions. You'll get the most out of medical school if you are impelled by some sort of desire to help others and blessed with boundless curiosity. You'll need the maturity and memory to handle a large volume of sometimes tedious learning; the ability to get on with people from all walks of life and a genuine interest in them; and sufficient humility to cope cheerfully with being at the bottom of the medical hierarchy for five years. It helps if you are good at forging strong and sustaining friendships—you'll need them when times get hard—and if you have some sort of moral and ethical value system that enables you to cope with the accelerated experience of life's extremes (birth, death, pain, suicide, suffering) that you will get during medical school.

REMEMBER

- Academic ability is not the only quality needed to secure a place at medical school.

- Broader attributes, such as compassion, endurance, determination, communication skills, enthusiasm, intellectual curiosity, balance, adaptability, integrity and a sense of humour are also needed.

- There are national guidelines regarding health and personal requirements to which all applicants must adhere. Failure to disclose information which may put patients at risk will result in losing a place at medical school.

- UK universities require ABB or higher at A level at first attempt, but this alone does not guarantee admission.

- A level chemistry (or physical science) is normally required but practically all of the medical schools will accept AS chemistry in its place. Biology is becoming the next preferred subject. All medical schools will accept at least one non-science A level.

- Scottish Highers and European/International Baccalaureate examinations are accepted at UK universities.

- Entry requirements for graduate applicants are more flexible, and options exist for some graduates to apply for shortened courses in some schools.

- Applicants who are resitting A levels will usually only be considered in special circumstances and should expect to be given higher entry requirements.

4. Choosing a medical school

The attitude that "beggars can't be choosers" is not only pessimistic but wrong. If, after serious consideration, you have decided that medicine is the right career for you and you are the right person for medicine, then the next step is to find a place at which to study where you can be happy and successful. This chapter is designed to help guide you into choosing the right schools to consider flirting with, rather than necessarily ending up (metaphorically speaking, of course) in bed with.

Walk into any medical school in the country and ask a bunch of the students which is the best medical school in the country and you will receive an almost universal shout of "This one, of course!" The general public's typical image of medical students is one of a group of young people who live life to the full, work hard, and play harder; hotheaded youngsters who can be excused their puerile pranks and mischievous misdemeanors, because, "Well, they must have a release from all that pressure, mustn't

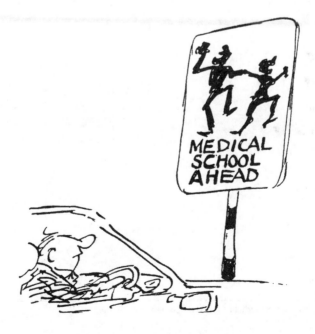

they". While this image should be treated with the same caution that is required with any stereotype, it none the less contains grains of truth. When you further consider the outstanding abilities of many medical students in their chosen extracurricular interests, it will come as no surprise to find that medical schools are full of students letting their hair down, getting involved in the things they enjoy, having a good time, and still doing enough work to pass those dreaded exams and assessments—or at least most of the time anyway. The only dilemma you have is to find which of these centres of social excitement and intellectual challenge best suits your particular interests and nature. Like all the best decisions in life the only way to find out is to do a bit of groundwork and research, plan out the lay of the land, then follow your instincts and go for it.

Medical schools vary greatly in the size of their yearly intake (Table 4.1). It is difficult to offer more precise advice about discovering the "spirit" or "identity" of an institution. However hard it may be to define, all the

Table 4.1—Predicted size of entry to first year of medicine in UK medical schools for 2003

Over 350
  Birmingham
  Leicester–Warwick
  King's (Guy's, King's and St Thomas')*

Over 300
  Liverpool
  Imperial
  Queen Mary's (Bart's and Royal London)
  UCL (Royal Free and University College)
  Manchester*
  Newcastle*
  Nottingham

Over 200
  Bristol*
  Cambridge
  Leeds
  St George's
  Sheffield*
  Edinburgh*
  Glasgow
  UWCM, Cardiff*

150–200
  Oxford
  Peninsula
  Southampton
  Aberdeen
  Dundee*
  Queen's, Belfast*

Less than 150
  Brighton–Sussex
  Hull–York
  East Anglia
  St Andrew's

---

*Indicates that a premedical (1st MB) course is available.

medical schools possess a uniqueness of which they are rightly proud. Of course some schools wear their hearts more on their sleeves than others or have a more easily identifiable image, but often the traditional identities are past memories, especially in London, where medical schools' identities have changed considerably in the past decade, particularly with recent amalgamations between medical schools and their mergers with larger multidisciplinary university colleges.

In days gone by a choice had to be made between a hospital based medical school, such as several in London, or an initially firmly multifaculty university environment, with a much broader student community with greater diversity of personalities, outlooks, and opportunities. This distinction has largely now disappeared; soon only the course at St George's in London will be hospital and medical school based throughout.

Accommodation may play an important part in choice, as some colleges house all the medics in one hall of residence while others spread them out, so you may end up living on a corridor with a lawyer, a historian, a musician, a dentist, a physicist, and someone who seems to sleep all day and smoke funny smelling tobacco who is allegedly doing "Media Studies and Ancient Icelandic".

Many find this kind of variety gives them exactly what they came to university for and would find spending all their work and play time with people on the same course socially stifling. While it is essentially a matter of personal preference, it is also worth noting that both have pros and cons—for example, when the workload is heavy it may be easier to knuckle down if everyone around you is doing likewise. Conversely when a bunch of medics get together they inevitably talk medicine, and, although recounting tales and anecdotes can amuse many a dinner party it may well breed narrow individuals with a social circle limited only to other medics. Choosing a campus site or a city site where you live side by side with the community your hospital serves may also have a different appeal.

Increasing diversity is being introduced to the design of the curriculum and how it is delivered. The traditional method of spending two or three years studying the basic sciences in the isolation of the medical school and never seeing a patient until you embarked on the clinical part of the course has all but disappeared. The teaching of subjects is generally much more integrated both between the different departments and between clinical and preclinical aspects. Even so, some curriculums are predominantly "systems based" and others "clinical problem based". Much more emphasis is being placed in all courses on clinical relevance, self directed learning and problem solving rather than memorising facts given in didactic lectures. There is substantial variation in the extent to which these changes have evolved and in many respects there is greater choice between courses than ever before. Diversity of approach is a strength of the United Kingdom system: "You pay your money and take your choice".

The courses at Oxford, Cambridge, and St Andrews remain more traditional in structure if not in subject matter and teaching methods.

These courses maintain a distinct separation between the more scientific and the more clinical, although they have moved away to some extent from separate subjects towards systems based teaching of the sciences and have introduced reference to clinical relevance; their philosophy is that it is still valid to study in depth the sciences related to medicine (anatomy, physiology, biochemistry, pharmacology, and pathology) as disciplines important in their own right, primarily as tools of intellectual development and scientific education rather than of vocational equipment. Cambridge and Oxford, however, have also introduced a four year course for graduate students, which combines the intellectual rigour of the traditional course with community-based clinical insights from the outset.

At Oxford all the basic sciences required for the professional qualifications are covered in the intensive first five terms' work and are then examined in the first BM. All students then take in their remaining four terms the honours school in physiology, a course much wider than its name suggests with options to choose from all the basic medical sciences, including pathology and psychology.

Cambridge adopts a more flexible approach. All the essential components of the medical sciences course are covered in two years. The third year is spent studying in depth one of a number of subjects, the choice being determined partly by whether or not the student is going on to continue a conventional clinical course at another university, usually, but not exclusively, London or Oxford, or continue on to the shorter Cambridge clinical course. For students remaining in Cambridge for clinical studies, the third year choices are limited to subjects approved by the GMC as "a year of medical study"; apart from the normal basic sciences these include subjects such as anthropology, history of medicine, social and political sciences, and zoology. Those moving on to a conventional clinical course have the attractive opportunity to spend their third year reading for a part II in any subject—law, music, or whatever takes their fancy—provided they have a suitable educational background and their local education authority is sufficiently inspired to support them. The three years lead to an honours BA.

At St Andrews the students spend three years studying for an ordinary degree or four years for an honours degree in medical sciences. Although strongly science based, clinical relevance is emphasised and some clinical insights are given, mainly in a community setting. Most St Andrews graduates go on to clinical studies at Manchester University, but a few go to other universities.

With the recent expansion in medical school places, the government has approved four completely new undergraduate medical schools. The first two of these—Peninsula Medical School (Universities of Exeter and Plymouth) and the University of East Anglia—started their first students on a standard five year course in Autumn 2002. Two further schools, Hull–York Medical School and Brighton and Sussex Medical School, will have their first students in Autumn 2003.

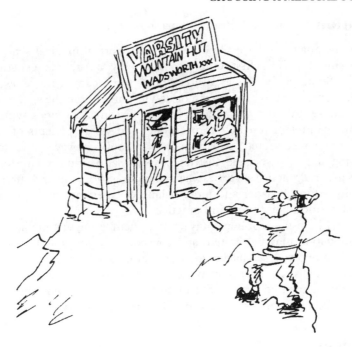

This then brings us back to those important but less tangible attractions of each medical school—the spirit and identity of the place. Unless you are an aficionado of architecture and simply could not concentrate unless in a neoclassical style lecture theatre or an art deco dissecting room, then what gives a place its unique character are the people who inhabit it; the biomedical science teachers, the hospital consultants who involve themselves in student life, the mad old dear who runs the canteen, the porter who knows everyone's name and most people's business, the all important dean and admissions tutor, and not least by any means the students themselves. It is the ever changing student body that above all else shapes the identity of a school and certainly gives it spirit and expresses its ever changing nature in a dynamic spirit. Just listen to any final year student bemoaning how the old place has changed and how the new first year just aren't the same as the rest of us and how what used to be like a rugby academy is more like a ballet school these days. What these oldies don't realise is that exactly the same was said five years ago when they were the freshers and five years before that and so on and so on.

The most obvious expression of this spirit is the plethora of clubs and societies that grow up in every medical school. Whatever your fancy it is worth investigating what facilities could be on offer. There is little point in being determined to gain entry to a medical school to pursue your hobby in climbing mountains if there is no tradition of such activities at that college, especially when another equally good college in other respects has a climbing wall on campus, a mountaineering hut in the Lake District, and an alpine club which goes on annual trips to Switzerland.

Location

Most individuals will have some idea of what sort of medical school they are looking for. The first criterion is usually a suitable geographical location. Some prefer to stay nearer home, some cannot move away fast enough. Some want to be up north or down south, out in the sticks or right in the smoke. Almost all medical schools are in large cities within the academic centres of research and teaching and where patients of endless variety are concentrated. Most medical schools, however, are making increasing use of associated district hospitals and primary care centres, such as general practice surgeries, in surrounding suburban and rural areas. This allows for a broader and more balanced experience and exposure to different medical conditions and practices.

If you wish to stay near home it is worth remembering that medical school accommodation may be limited, and consequently you may be given low priority and find yourself having to live at home. The downside is that those not living in halls of residence with their new friends and having to commute to and from home find it more difficult to immerse themselves in student life and may end up feeling isolated and unfulfilled by university life.

Finances

An increasingly important issue related to accommodation and other living costs which has to be considered is student debt. Surveys over the past 10 years have shown a consistent and alarming rise in the levels of debt for all students, in both the government student loans scheme and in overdrafts and loans from banks. The situation is worse for medical students because of the length of the course, the shorter vacations in the later years, and the intensive nature of the training and exams limiting opportunities for part time casual work. Other factors such as expensive books and equipment and the need to dress appropriately also add to the cost; turning up to the professor's clinic attired in smelly old trainers, ragged jeans, and an "I love Britney" T-shirt is hardly portraying a professional image.

The one advantage that medical students do have over many other students is that when they qualify they are pretty certain of falling into secure and reasonably well paid jobs. Still, seeing a large chunk of your hard earned first pay cheque disappear into the repayments of your several thousand pound debt is not a pleasant feeling, especially when the shackles of debt can last for several years after you leave medical school. The size of individuals' debts at the end of their time at medical school can vary enormously, depending on personal circumstances, but it is now not uncommon for students to owe at least £10 000, and in many cases considerably more. For overseas students who do not qualify for student loans and who have to pay full tuition fees, most schools expect proof of the ability not only to pay the fees but also of resources to live on during their time at medical school.

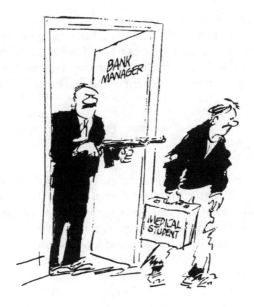

For mature students, particularly graduates, who may not qualify for the usual support from their local council, the Departments of Health for England and Wales now have a bursary scheme to support the last three years of training. The amounts which will be paid vary according to the student's individual case, for instance if they have children to support or other income sources. More information can be obtained by reading *Financial Help for Healthcare Students* (5th edition) (which is available online at www.doh.gov.uk/hcsmain.htm) or by contacting NHS Careers (tel 0845 6060655).

It would be sensible then to consider that in choosing your medical school some areas are obviously more expensive to live in than others. It should not, however, completely put you off these areas because many students in London or Edinburgh, for instance, believe that the advantages they have of being in such a place are well worth the extra expense. It is therefore worth finding out about the cost and availability of accommodation and general living expenses at any school that you are keen on.

Range of entrance requirements

Choice of medical school must be guided by a realistic expectation of the chances of achieving its basic entrance requirements. This does not just mean will you reach the right grades, all of which are between ABB and AAA for A levels but, more importantly, have you done acceptable subjects, and acceptable exams (see pp. 27–29).

Overseas students from outside the European Union should check with medical authorities in their own country which medical schools will provide them with a qualification that will be recognised at home, as not all

United Kingdom medical degrees may be acceptable. Overseas students should check the quota allowed for each school and whether any particular criteria are used in selecting applicants—for example, if priority is given to students from the developing world or countries with historic links to one school or another or to students without a medical school in their own country.

A gap year?

Most schools now encourage students to take a gap year if they want to, although it is not a requirement. It is important however to follow some basic ground rules. Firstly, if you are planning a gap year, ensure you mark your UCAS form for deferred entry. Although you can apply for this retrospectively, it is much more likely that schools will agree to your request if they know about it as early as possible. Secondly, have some firm plans of what you want to do in your year out and why. It is something you should write—albeit briefly—in your personal statement and is a common topic for questioning in an interview. Your year out does not need to be spent doing anything medical, but you may want it to be, nor does it always have to involve travelling to the four corners of the earth. Finally, it is worth remembering that five or six years at medical school for most people means a considerable financial debt. So if you can spend some time earning some money, it will certainly come in useful; whatever you do, do not start your course already burdened with a large overdraft and credit card bills. Most of all, enjoy your gap year; it will give you lots of experiences you will never forget and be a great preparation for life as a student.

Mature and graduate students

A considerable number of graduates and other mature students decide medicine is for them. UCAS uses a definition of being 21 years of age or over as being "mature" for the basis of medical school applications. Trying to find a medical school presents them with many of the same challenges and choices that face school leavers, but with added problems on top. Family or personal commitments may limit the choice of geographical location of a school. Financial commitments such as mortgages and reduced income will also affect mature students' choices. These factors, however, must be set against the government's commitment to attracting medical students from more diverse educational and socioeconomic backgrounds, and the recent rapid expansion in available places for this purpose. In addition an increasing number of medical schools are introducing shortened courses for students with science or healthcare related degrees. In the next few years, many medical schools are planning such moves although the numbers of available places and the precise nature of graduates they are designed for will vary from school to school.

Practically all schools are happy to consider applications from mature students, but it is fair to say that successful applicants over 30 are unusual—though there are some notable exceptions—and medical students over 40 are very rare. Schools tend not to have specific quotas but will judge each case on merit, although in the past mature students have counted for about 10 per cent on conventional courses. Some schools have better records of admitting mature students than others, and some actually encourage such applications in their prospectus (for example Leeds, Manchester, Southampton, St George's, and Guy's, King's & St Thomas').

The schools which currently offer shortened course for graduates (usually, but not exclusively, in life science or related subjects) include Birmingham, Dundee, Leicester–Warwick, Newcastle, St George's, Oxford, and Cambridge. Bart's and the Royal London and Cardiff currently have shortened courses for dental graduates who wish to pursue maxillo-facial surgery.

Several other schools are planning similar courses for entry in Autumn 2003 or 2004 including Aberdeen, Liverpool, Nottingham, Imperial College, Royal Free and University College, Southampton, and University of Wales (joint venture between Cardiff and Swansea). It is worth checking up-to-date details with these schools nearer the time for application as they are changing all the time and some are still awaiting formal approval of their courses and funding arrangements. Also the numbers of available places vary from school to school and year to year, as do their selection criteria and the precise design of their curriculum. For example, at Cambridge, arts graduates are particularly encouraged in the expectation that they may bring a different perspective and that through the college system they will receive the necessary academic and pastoral support. Three Cambridge colleges are sharing the responsibility for these students: Hughes Hall, Lucy Cavendish (women only), and Wolfson. Arts graduates are expected to have acquired basic science knowledge, whether through A levels or an approved foundation course. St George's requires satisfactory performance in a professionally designed written entrance exam testing basic knowledge, reasoning skills, and communication.

This variety is increasing choices for prospective medical students, and means you will need to shop around to find what suits you best.

Interview or no interview

If you have a fear of interviews or an objection to being selected on the basis of an interview then there are schools which still do not interview (Table 4.2), despite the trend towards more schools adopting the interview as a useful adjunct to the confidential reference, the academic record, and the student's own comments on the UCAS form.

Table 4.2—Interviewing policies of United Kingdom medical schools according to whether or not they normally interview shortlisted applicants

Medical school	Interviews
Birmingham	Yes
Brighton and Sussex	Yes
Bristol	Yes
Cambridge	Yes
East Anglia	Yes
Hull–York	Yes
Leeds	Yes
Leicester–Warwick	Yes
Liverpool	Yes
Imperial College, London	Yes
King's College, London (Guy's, King's and St Thomas')	Yes
Queen Mary and Westfield College, London (Bart's and Royal London)	Yes
St George's, London	Yes
University College, London (Royal Free and University College)	Yes
Manchester	Yes
Newcastle	Yes
Nottingham	Yes
Oxford	Yes
Peninsula	Yes
Sheffield	Yes
Southampton	No, only interview non-school leavers
Aberdeen	Yes, but not in all cases
Dundee	Yes
Edinburgh	No, only interview non-school leavers
Glasgow	Yes
St Andrew's	No
University of Wales, Cardiff	Yes
Queen's University, Belfast	No

Visits and open days

In summary, there are numerous factors which prospective students should take into consideration when deciding which medical schools to apply to, some relevant to all students and some specific to special cases. The most important advice is to visit as many schools as possible, take in the general feel of the place, look at the accommodation and facilities, explore the local area, and especially take time to talk to the current students, most of whom will, of course, be biased in favour of their school but who will at least be able to enthuse about the good points and answer your questions. Open days and sixth form conferences provide a more formal opportunity to do this. Later, a visit for interview may reinforce first impressions. A little careful groundwork can not only improve your chances of obtaining a place at a medical school but also help you to ensure that that place is at the right school in which to spend some of the best years of your life.

REMEMBER

- Medical schools vary greatly in size, location and style.

- Most, but not all, medical schools are in large cities, but often use hospitals and health centres in nearby towns and villages for teaching attachments.

- Cost of living can vary considerably between different parts of the country.

- Availability and quality of accommodation and leisure facilities should be considered.

- Living at home costs less, but most students prefer to move away from home and widen their experience.

- Courses are all giving increasing emphasis to clinical relevance and experience in the early years, but some have more than others.

- Only one school—St George's—is entirely hospital campus based throughout.

- Check up on the medical school's attitude to overseas students and mature applicants if relevant to you.

- Many opportunities now exist for graduates to apply for shortened courses.

- Most importantly do your homework—read the prospectuses (most universities publish an official one and an "alternative prospectus" written by students), read the online prospectus or course outline and selection criteria on the school's website, attend open days, careers fairs or ring medical schools to arrange to look round—most will be happy to oblige—you can get a feel for the place, check out the facilities, and you will be able to ask questions of students already there.

5. Application and selection

The whole emphasis of this book is to aid and encourage potential medical students to examine properly the career they are considering. This chapter deals in more detail with some of the practical "nuts and bolts" of the process of applying to and being selected by a medical school. All too often careers advice concentrates too much on these practicalities, implying the only criteria for choosing future doctors are whether they can fill out an impressive application form and get themselves selected. This detracts from the more important process of your addressing medicine's suitability as a career for you, and your suitability to be a doctor. Only after giving this serious consideration should you consider the details of application and selection set out in this chapter.

Unfortunately, the qualities which count for most in medicine are not precisely measurable. The measurable—examination performance at school—neither necessarily relates to these qualities nor guarantees intellectual or practical potential. Stewart Wolfe, an American physician, was right to ask:

> Are the clearly specified and hence readily defensible criteria those most likely to yield a wise and cultivated doctor—a person capable of dealing with uncertainty, of compassionate understanding and wise judgment? Can an ideal physician be expected from an intellectual *forme fuste* who has spent his college years only learning the "right answers"?

Furthermore, there is no acceptable objective measure of the quality of the doctor against which to test the validity of selection decisions. In this sea of uncertainty it is not surprising that selection processes are open to criticism. None the less, few patients would choose a doctor without meeting him or her first and a strong argument can be made for discovering the people behind their UCAS forms, if only briefly. Also, many applicants think that they should have a opportunity to put their own case for becoming a doctor.

Selection for interview (and at some schools for offer without interview) is made on the strength of an application submitted through UCAS. An application completed partly by the applicant and partly by a referee, usually the head or a member of the school staff, who submits a confidential reference.

Altogether, about 12 000 home and European Union applicants compete for over 6000 (soon to be 7000) places to read medicine at United Kingdom universities, together with about 1500 overseas students who compete for about 330 places. Women comprise over half of all applicants and entrants. Some of the new places are on new accelerated courses for graduates (see p. 40).

It is worth completing the UCAS form accurately and legibly. Deans and admission tutors who have to scan a thousand or two application forms (which they receive reduced in size from the original application) simply do not have time to spend deciphering illegible handwriting. A legible, even stylish, presentation creates a good impression from the start.

Personal details

The first section of the UCAS form presents the personal details of the applicant, including age on 30 September of the coming academic year. Many applicants give instead their current age and at a glance seem to fall below the minimum age for entry at some medical schools or to be so young that older applicants might reasonably be given priority over them. True, the date of birth is also requested, but the quickly scanning eye may not pick up the discrepancy.

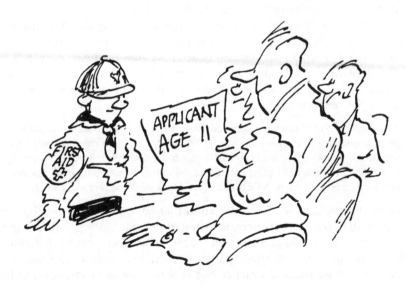

The list of schools attended by an applicant is often a useful guide to the educational opportunity received. More ability and determination are needed to emerge as a serious candidate for medicine from an unselective school with

2000 pupils, of whom only 10–15 normally enter university each year, than from a selective school for which university entry is the norm.

Choices

Applicants are not expected to give all their course choices to medicine. Six university courses can be nominated on UCAS forms, and the medical schools have requested that applicants should limit the number of applications for medicine to four. The remaining choices can be used for an alternative course without prejudice to the applications for medicine. You should remember, however, that if a backup offer for a non-medical course is accepted and the candidate fails to get the grades for medical school but does sufficiently well for the backup then that offer has to be accepted, and it is not possible to enter clearing for medicine. The only alternative is to withdraw from university entry in that year and to apply again the following year.

Other information

Examination results should be clearly listed by year. It is sensible to list first those subjects immediately relevant to the science requirements for medicine and those subjects needed for university matriculation, usually English language and mathematics. All attempts at examinations should be entered and clearly separated. The date and number of A level or degree examinations yet to be taken complete the picture.

While it probably never pays to try to amuse on an application form it is worth being interesting. Your personal statement presents an opportunity to catch the eye of a tired admissions dean because medicine demands so much more than academic ability, so include mention of your outside interests and experiences. John Todd, a consultant physician, observed from his own experience that:

> The value of the physician is derived far more from what may be called his general qualities than from his special knowledge ... such qualities as good judgment, the ability to see a patient as a whole, the ability to see all aspects of a problem in the right perspective and the ability to weigh up evidence are far more important than the detailed knowledge of some rare syndrome.

Small details, such as the information that an applicant spends his free moments delivering newspapers, assisting in the village shop, and acting as "pall-bearer and coffin-carrier to the local undertaker" converts a cipher into a person. None of those particular activities may be immediately relevant to future medical practice but at least they show initiative. Other activities, such as hobbies, music, drama, and sport, indicate a willingness and ability to acquire intellectual and practical skills and to participate, characteristics useful in life in general but also to a medical school which needs its own cultural life to divert tired minds and to develop full personalities during a long course of training.

Some applicants offer a remarkably wide variety of accomplishments, such as the boy who declared in his UCAS form: "I play various types of music, including jazz, Irish traditional, orchestral and military band, on trombone, fiddle, tin whistle, mandolin, and bodhran. ... " If Irish music be the food of medicine, play on. But that was not all, for he continued: "I also enjoy boxing and I have a brown belt (judo). My more social pastimes include ballroom dancing, photography, driving and motor cycling." Would this young man have time for medicine?

It is not sensible to enter every peripheral interest and pastime lest it appears, as indeed may be so, that many of these activities are superficial. It is also unwise for an applicant to enter any interest that he or she would be unable to discuss intelligently at interview.

The applicant's own account of interests and the confidential report (for which a whole page is available) sometimes bring to life the different sides of an applicant's character. For example, one young man professed "a great interest in music" and confessed that he was "lead vocalist in a rowdy pop group" while his headmaster reported that he was "fairly quiet in lessons ... science and medicine afford him good motivation ... his choice of career suits him well. There is no doubt that he has the ability and temperament successfully to follow his calling". All in all this interplay of information is useful, for medicine is a suitable profession for multifaceted characters.

The confidential report is always important and is sometimes crucial. Most teachers take great care to give a balanced, realistic assessment of progress and potential in these confidential reports. Readers of UCAS forms quickly discover the few schools pupilled entirely by angels. Cautionary nuances are more commonly conveyed by what is omitted than by what is said, but a few heads are sufficiently outspoken to write from the hip in appropriate circumstances. Euphemisms may or may not be translated such as: "Economy of effort and calm optimism have been the hall mark of his academic process. Put another way, his teachers used to complain of idleness and lack of interest." Others indicate that they are attempting to get the candidate to come to terms with reality. For example: "We have explained to him that you are not in the business to supply fairy tale endings to touching UCAS references and that you will judge him on his merits."

It sounded as if that candidate was likely to come to the same fate as the would be officer cadet rejected from Sandhurst with the explanation that "he sets himself extremely low standards—unfortunately he totally fails to live up to them". Not that every head gets it right, like the one whose pen slipped in writing, "Ian also has the distinction of being something of an expert in breeding erotic forms of rabbits".

Fair but frank confidential references are an essential part of an acceptable selection process. The confidential report usually includes a prediction of performance at A level, useful because it is set in the context of the report as a whole; but predictions can be misleading. A recent survey of the accuracy of A level predictions indicated that only about one third turned out to be correct, a half were too high (and half of these by two or more grades) and a tenth were too low. Occasionally a candidate is seriously underestimated, with the result that an interview is not offered and the applicant is at the mercy of the clearing procedure after the results are declared or has to apply again next year. Application to medical school after the results are known would be fairer but the practical difficulties in changing the system have so far proved insuperable.

Getting an interview

What in the mass of information counts most in the decision to shortlist a candidate for interview or even, at some medical schools, an offer without interview? Grades achieved in GCSE and A level if already taken or predicted grades if not yet taken are universally important. Medical schools also take notice of, but may give different weighting to, outstanding achievement in any field because excellence is not lightly achieved. They look for evidence of determination, perseverance, and consideration for others; for an ability to communicate, for breadth and depth of other interests, especially to signs of originality, for the contribution likely to be made to the life of the medical school, for a solid confidential report, and for assessment of potential for further development by taking all the evidence together. Highly though achievement is valued, potential, both personal and intellectual, is even more important. Perceptive shortlisters look for applicants who are just beginning to get into their stride in preference to those who have already been forced to their peak, aptly described by Dorothy L Sayers in *Gaudy Night* as possessed of "small summery brains that flower early and run to seed". Although the shortlisting process deliberately sets out to view applicants widely, analysis of the outcome has shown that academic achievement still carries the weight in selecting candidates from their UCAS forms. The great majority of applicants called for interview are academically strong, and it is then that their personal characteristics decide the outcome (see next chapter).

What weight is put on medically related work experience in shortlisting—and what indeed is "medically related"? If you look through the stated views of individual medical schools in the *UCAS Guide to Entry to Medicine* on the "qualities" they are seeking in applicants, you will find three constantly recurring themes: communication skills, evidence of concern for the welfare of others, and a realistic perception of what medicine entails. It follows that any work experience that entails dealing with the public, actively helping or caring for others, or which shows doctors at work and health care in action may enable you to be convincing in establishing your ability to communicate, your understanding of what you would be letting yourself in for, and your discovery of the skills and attributes you already possess which make you suitable in principle for the responsibilities of a doctor. It is not so much precisely what you do but why you have done it and what you have both given to it and gained from it.

Applicants could legitimately ask whether any factors, apart from the strength of the UCAS application form, enter into the selection for interview. It used to be customary at many medical schools (a tradition by no means confined to them) for the children of graduates of the school or of staff to be offered an interview, but that has now been abandoned out of conviction that the selection process must be and be seen to be open and, as far as can be, scrupulously fair.

Unsolicited letters of recommendation are a sensitive matter. Factual information additional to the UCAS confidential report is occasionally important and is welcome from any source. For example, one applicant had left another medical school in his first term against the advice of his dean to work to support his mother and younger brother. Three years later, when the family was on its feet and he wanted to reapply to medical school, he was under a cloud for having given up his place. The UCAS form did not tell the full story; and a note from the family doctor was most helpful in giving the full background to a courageous and self sacrificing young man. Some other unsolicited letters add only the information that an applicant is either well connected or has good friends, and it is difficult to see why such applicants should be given an advantage over those whose friends do not feel it proper to canvass.

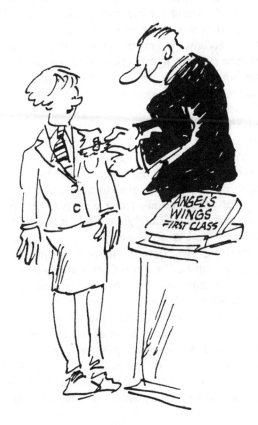

It is not only unsolicited testimonials that recommend in glowing terms. How could any dean resist the angel described thus by her headmaster:

> The charm of her personal character defies analysis. She is possessed by all the graces and her noble qualities impress everybody. She has proved the soul of courtesy and overlying all her virtues is sound common sense. She has always been mindful of her obligations and has fulfilled her responsibilities and duties as a prefect admirably well. Amiable and industrious, she appears to have a spirit incapable of boredom and her constructive loyalty to the school, along with her unfailing good nature, has won her the high esteem and admiration of staff and contemporaries alike. We recommend her warmly as a top drawer student.

A "top drawer" student indeed—and a top drawer headmaster.

When to apply

All UCAS forms for applicants to medicine must be received by 15 October at the latest, so get on with it as early as possible. Late applications are rarely even considered and almost never successful.

In principle a year's break between school and university is a good thing. The year is particularly valuable if used to experience the discipline and, often, the drudgery of earning a living from relatively unskilled work. It can provide insights for students (most of whom come from relatively well off families) into the everyday life and thinking of the community which will provide most of their patients in due course and may be very different from their own background. There is no need for such work to be in the setting of health care; in fact much is to be said for escaping from the environment of doctors and hospitals.

If the earnings of these months are then used to discover something of different cultures abroad that is a bonus. Alternatively, you may work abroad through Project Trust, Gap Projects, Operation Raleigh, or other similar organisations. But just being a year older, more experienced, and more mature is, in itself, helpful to the discipline and motivation of study and especially useful when you are faced with patients. In practice, short term employment may, unfortunately, be difficult to find but there are few places where work of some description cannot be obtained if a student is prepared to do anything legal, however menial. Settling down to academic work again after a year off can be a problem, but it is not insuperable if the motivation and self discipline are there. If commitment has evaporated after a year's break, better to have discovered early than late; better to drop out before starting rather than to waste a place that another could use and to waste your own time, which could better be channelled elsewhere.

A practical dilemma arises for those planning a year off over whether to apply for deferred entry before taking A levels or to apply with completed A levels early the year afterwards. Universities may be reluctant to commit themselves a year ahead to average applicants because the standard seems to be rising all the time. Outstanding applicants, however, should have no difficulty in arranging deferred entry before taking A levels, but it is worth checking the policy of schools in which you are interested before application. If you are not offered a deferred place apply early the next year and send a covering letter to the deans of your chosen medical schools asking for as early an interview as possible if you are planning to go abroad.

REMEMBER

- Each year about 12 000 home and EU students apply for 6000 (soon to be 7000) places to read medicine in the UK.

- Some of the additional places will be shorter courses for graduates, mostly, but not entirely, science graduates.

- About 1500 overseas students compete for 330 reserved places.

- Women comprise just over half of applicants and entrants.

- Academic achievement is the strongest determinant in selection, but broader interests and achievements also count.

- It generally pays to apply as early as possible.

- Applications should be legible, honest, and, as far as possible, interesting.

- Use four choices for medicine; it is entirely reasonable to give a fifth and sixth to a non-medical option, but this is not compulsory.

- If you are planning a gap year, apply for a deferred entry rather than delay your application, and be prepared to discuss your plans for the year at interview.

6. Interviews

Academics and careers advisers may argue about the usefulness and fairness of an interview in the process for selecting future medical students and doctors. Those on the receiving end—the candidates—are unanimous in the belief that the interview is somewhere between daunting and dreadful. Some of the dread is fear of the unknown, as well as fear of being judged on what is little more than first impressions. Read on, and you may have some of those fears dispelled and be able to give yourself a better chance at creating a positive impression.

On a dull overcast day due for an imminent downpour, you step off the early morning train in your best new outfit, shoes polished, hair neatly brushed, clutching a copy of a newspaper in which you have just been reading an article about trendy new treatments for anxiety. As you approach the gates of the medical school and see the sign directing "Interview Candidates This

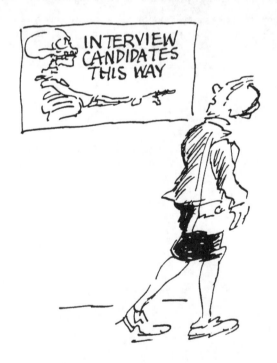

Way" you wish you could remember any of the useful tips from that newspaper article; as it is you are so nervous you are no longer sure you can even remember your own name. It is not your first interview for a place at medical school, you had one last week. Although most of the details are lost in a haze of pounding heartbeats and sweaty palms, you are unable to rid yourself of the image of that professor's face when you dug yourself into a hole discussing the nutritional requirements of the Twa pygmies, a subject in which the sum of your knowledge was gleaned from the last five minutes of a late night documentary on BBC2. In what seemed like only half a minute, you are back at the railway station, on your way home, while the fearsome trio of interviewers dissect your inner being and decide your worth for that precious place at their medical school; your passport to their worthy profession. It feels like your life is in their hands.

SS

Most medical schools interview those students who seem the strongest on paper (through past achievements, predicted exam success, the confidential reference, and the student's own statements on the application form) and use the 15 to 20 minute interview as a way of choosing between them. The remaining schools interview smaller numbers such as mature students, in an attempt to assess motivation and circumstances more fully (see Table 4.2, p. 42).

The purpose

In general the interview is an opportunity to test the students' awareness of what they are letting themselves in for, both at medical school and as a doctor, ranging from the impact of medicine on personal life to how medicine relates to the society it serves. It also allows the interviewers to explore whether applicants can communicate effectively, can think a problem through with logic and reason, and are speaking for themselves and not regurgitating well rehearsed answers which teachers and parents have thought up for them; it also reveals some of the qualities above and beyond academic ability which are desirable in a caring profession, such as compassion and a sense of humour. Occasionally a student who seems outstanding on paper can seem so lacking in motivation, insight, or humanity that he or she loses an offer which would otherwise have seemed a certainty. Likewise the interview can allow students who seem equal on their UCAS forms to make their own case either through special circumstances or by a shining performance.

The panel

The interview panels differ in style and substance between schools but typically consist of three or four members of staff and often a student. The panel is a mixture of basic scientists, hospital consultants, and general practitioners, one of whom, often the dean or admissions tutor, will take the chair. Members of panels attend in an individual capacity and not as representatives of particular specialties. They know that medicine offers a wide range of career opportunities, that most doctors will end up looking after patients but not all do, that more will work outside hospitals than in, and that both the training and the job itself are demanding physically and emotionally. They also know that whatever their final occupation doctors need to make decisions, deal with uncertainty, and communicate effectively and compassionately with patients and colleagues alike as well as maintaining moderately exacting academic standards. The aim is not to pick men and women for specific tasks but to train wise, bright, humane, rounded individuals who will find their niche somewhere in medicine. The format may be formal, with the interview conducted in traditional fashion across a large table, or more informal, sitting in comfortable chairs around a coffee table by the fireside. The tenor of the interview, however, depends much more on the style of questioning; no matter how soft the armchairs are, they can still feel decidedly uncomfortable if you are made to feel like you are being grilled and about to be eaten for breakfast.

Dress and demeanour

Although the interview is a chance to be yourself and sell yourself, there are certain codes of conduct that even the most individual or eccentric candidate should be encouraged to heed. Rightly or wrongly first impressions count, and so what you wear matters. Dress smartly and comfortably and make an effort to look as presentable as you would expect from a mature professional. If your usual style of clothing is rather off beat, then perhaps for once it may be wise to let your tongue make any statements about your individuality rather than your all in one leather number and preference for nose piercing.

Nothing is more of a turn off to interviewers than someone who is full of himself (or herself!) and seems to be finding it hard to accept that his offer is not a formality. On the other hand an obviously talented and caring student whose modesty and nerves get the better of him and who fails to give the panel any reasons at all to give him an offer is almost as frustrating. The key is balance. When asked to blow your own trumpet make it sound like a melodious fugue not a ship's fog horn. The best way to learn how to achieve this delicate balance is by practice. Many schools will be able to organise mock interviews, which can be useful, but often the more specific points relating to entering medical school can be best thought through by enlisting the help of your local family doctor or a family friend who is a doctor or by talking to anyone experienced in interviewing or being interviewed in any context or by asking the advice of people who have themselves recently been through it when you visit the medical schools on open days or tours.

The conversation

Almost anything can be asked. It would be advisable to have thought about such things as why medicine? why here? why now? You should be able to show you have a realistic insight into the life of a doctor, and this is often best achieved by relating personal experience of spending some time with a doctor in hospital or general practice or, for example, by voluntary work in an old people's home or with children with special needs. Some panels put great store by your showing them how much you can achieve when you put your mind to it and will want to discuss your expedition to Nepal, your work on the school magazine, your musical or sporting successes. Remember to keep a copy of your UCAS form personal statement to read before you go into your interview. It is very often used as a source for questions and it can be embarrassing if you appear not to remember what you wrote. Even more importantly, do not invent interests or experience, as you may get caught out. One candidate at interview recently struggled through his interview after he was asked about the voluntary work at a local nursing home which he put on his form and replied: "I haven't actually got round to doing it yet, but I'd like to." He was not offered a place.

It is often sensible to have kept in touch with current affairs and developments in research. This is particularly relevant if the medical school has a strong interest in a research topic which has a high media profile. By reading a good quality daily newspaper you will greatly assist your ability to provide informed comment on issues of the moment. One candidate at interview cited the strong research background as a reason for applying to that school, and when asked to discuss which research at the school impressed him he replied: "Fleming's discovery of penicillin". He knew he had not done himself any favours when the dean replied: "Could you not perhaps think of anything a little more recent than 1928?"

With contentious issues such as ethics or politics, candidates will be neither criticised nor penalised for holding particular views but will be expected to be capable of explaining their case. Specific questions on subjects such as abortion, religion, or party politics are discouraged, but if they are likely to cause personal professional dilemmas it is reasonable and sensible to have thought about them and to be able to discuss how you would approach resolving such issues. Candidates with special circumstances, especially mature students, should be fully prepared for the interview panel to concentrate on particularly relevant factors such as whether they can afford to support themselves during the course, rigorous testing of their motivation, and questioning of the reasons behind their decision to enter the medical profession.

It is usual for the panel to offer an opportunity for the candidate to ask questions. A current student at the school sitting in on the interview can often be useful in answering the candidate's questions. Make sure if you do ask a question that you do not spoil an otherwise successful interview by asking a question which simply indicates that you have failed to read the prospectus thoroughly or which has no direct bearing on your entry to or time at medical school.

Offers

An offer made to a candidate who has already achieved the minimum academic requirement is unconditional. All candidates who have already attained the minimum grades at first attempt cannot automatically receive a place because far more applicants will achieve this than the school can take. Offers are made on all round merit as can best be assessed on all the evidence.

If the A level examinations have yet to be taken an offer is conditional on the candidate achieving the required grades at first attempt. Occasionally a student who seems in need of an incentive may be given a higher target but would normally be accepted with the minimum. Sometimes a lower than normal offer is made to reduce the pressure on a candidate working under exceptional circumstances. If A levels are being retaken, most medical schools will expect higher than normal targets to be reached.

Finally, applicants must remember that achievement of minimum grades does no more than qualify them to enter the real competition. No level of examination success gives entitlement to a place without necessary consideration of the other factors important to being a doctor, an assessment of which is the whole basis for calling applicants to interview. Many more candidates can achieve the required grades than can possibly be taken under the fixed quota system which exists for the training of doctors. All medical schools try very hard to be fair but a number of able applicants will inevitably be disappointed.

REMEMBER

- Most medical schools interview all applicants to whom they make an offer.

- Usually a panel of three to five people—doctors, lecturers and often a student observer—will be present.

- The interview will usually last 10–20 minutes, giving you time to settle into it—the interviewers know that you will be nervous, but try to relax and show yourself at your best.

- The major purpose of an interview is to test your awareness about the course and the career, and to discover whether you can think and reason for yourself.

- To prepare for the day read the prospectus thoroughly, read up on current relevant issues in the health section of a daily newspaper, arrange some practice interviews and be prepared to elaborate on what you wrote on your application form.

- On the day dress smartly and comfortably, arrive in plenty of time, speak up clearly and do not ask questions that have no direct bearing on entry to, or time at, medical school.

- Offers will be unconditional if the academic requirements have already been met, or for most applicants will be conditional on achieving target grades at the first attempt.

- All medical schools try hard to be fair but some able applicants will inevitably be disappointed.

7. Medical school: the early years

The first few weeks at medical school are bewildering. On top of all the upheaval of finding your feet in a new place, finding new friends, finding the supermarket, and finding that your bed does not miraculously make itself, you will find yourself at the beginning of a course that will mould the rest of your life. Ahead there are new subjects to study, a whole new language to learn, a new approach to seeing problems, new experiences and challenges, thrills and spills, ups and downs, laughter and tears. You are now at university, you are a medical student and you are on your way to being a doctor.

Until recently the undergraduate medical course had remained largely unaltered for decades, having slowly and steadily evolved over centuries of medical learning. All that has had to change in the past decade as the structure of the traditional course came face to face with the strains of modern medicine. The explosion of scientific knowledge, the unstoppable advances in technology, the ever developing complexity of clinical practice, and changing health care provision have all added to the tremendous demands on tomorrow's doctors.

At the same time there has been a reaction against the soaring dominance of modern science over old-fashioned art in medicine, technical capability over wise restraint, and process over humanity. A growing concern (not necessarily justified) that preoccupation with the diagnostic and therapeutic potential of molecular biology will obscure the patient as a whole person, a person who so often simply does not feel well for relatively trivial and unscientific reasons, and probably only needs to be listened to and encouraged to take responsibility for his or her own health. A fear that healthcare teams under pressure from every direction may give the impression that they have forgotten how to care in the fullest sense—and, worse still, may indeed lose sight of the humanity of medicine.

The Prince of Wales put his finger on the issue in a "Personal View" in the *British Medical Journal*, writing "Many patients feel rushed and confused at seeing a different doctor each time … and many healthcare professionals feel frustrated and dissatisfied at being unable to deliver the quality of care they would like in today's overstretched service."

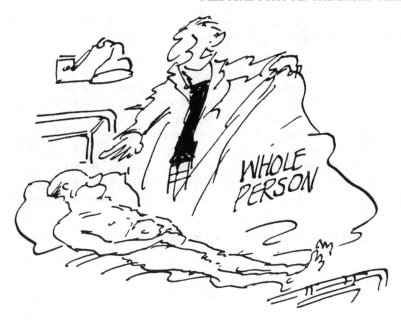

There has also been a reaction against the traditionally closed mind of the medical profession towards complementary and alternative medicine, partly because of dissatisfaction with the fragmentation of conventional medicine and partly because of the effects of relentless pressure on doctors. As some patients derive benefit from unorthodox medicine (often when traditional medicine has failed)—however obscure the mechanism of the benefit may be—doctors need to be informed about such therapies and the evidence, such as it is, for their effectiveness. As the Prince of Wales observed in his "Personal View": "It would be a tragic loss if traditional human caring had to move to complementary medicine, leaving orthodox medicine with just the technical management of disease". At the end of the day, it may well be that the greatest benefit of complementary therapies derives from the therapist being able to give more time to listening to the patient. Be that as it may, it is clearly in the patient's interest to "create a more inclusive system that incorporates the best and most effective of both complementary and orthodox medicine ... choice where appropriate, and the best of both worlds whenever it is possible."

Recommendations published by the GMC in 1993 (revised 2002) provided a new impetus to the introduction of a new medical curriculum. Less emphasis was put on absorbing facts like a sponge and more on thinking: on listening, analysing, questioning, problem solving, explaining, and involving the patient in his or her own care; more emphasis on the patient as a whole in his or her human setting. The biological and behavioural basis of medicine in most medical schools now focuses on "need to know and understand". Oxford and Cambridge remain perfectly reasonable exceptions, having retained a strongly and intrinsically medical science centred curriculum in the first three years. The GMC encourages diversity within the curriculum and students should carefully consider which sort of curriculum would best inspire their mind, heart, and enthusiasm.

You can usually get a flavour of how the course is delivered at each school by reading the curriculum and students' views section on the medical schools' websites or in their prospectuses.

Nevertheless, at most universities the traditionally separate scientific and clinical aspects of the course have become very substantially integrated to prevent excited and enthusiastic students becoming disillusioned in the first two years with what understandably seemed to be divorced from real patients and real lives, from clinical relevance and clinical understanding.

The subjects, systems, and topics

Most first year students begin with a foundation course covering the fundamental principles of the basic medical sciences. These include anatomy—the structure of the human body, including cell and tissue biology and embryology, the process of development; physiology—the normal functions of the body; biochemistry—the chemistry of body processes, with increasing amounts of molecular biology and genetics; pharmacology—the properties and metabolism of drugs within the body; psychology and sociology—the basis of human behaviour and the placing of health and illness in a wider context; and basic pathology—the general principles underlying the process of disease.

As the general understanding of the basics increases, the focus of the teaching often then moves from parallel courses in each individual subject to integrated interdepartmental teaching based on body systems—such as the respiratory system, the cardiovascular system, or the locomotor system—and into topics such as development and aging, infection and immunity, and public health and epidemiology.

In the systems approach the anatomy, physiology, and biochemistry of a system can be looked at simultaneously, building up knowledge of the body in a steady logical way. As time and knowledge progress the pathology and pharmacology of the system can be studied, and the psychological and sociological aspects of related illnesses are considered.

Often the normal structure and function can best be understood by illustrating how it can go wrong in disease, and so clinicians are increasingly involved at an early stage; this has an added advantage of placing the science into a patient focused context, making the subject more relevant and stimulating for would be doctors. It also allows for early contact with patients to take place in the form of clinical demonstrations or, for example, in a project looking at chronic disease in a general practice population or on a hospital ward.

In some medical schools, such as Manchester and Liverpool, practically all the learning in the early years is built around clinical problems that focus all the different dimensions of knowledge needed to understand the illness, the patient, and the management.

The teaching and the teachers

The teaching of these subjects usually takes the form of lectures, laboratory practicals, demonstrations, films, tutorials and projects, and, increasingly, computer assisted interactive learning programmes; even virtual reality is beginning to find its uses in teaching medical students.

The teaching of anatomy in particular has undergone great change. Dissection of dead bodies (cadavers) has been replaced in most schools by increased use of closed circuit television and demonstrations of prosected specimens and an ever improving range of synthetic models. Preserved cadavers make for difficult dissection, especially in inexperienced if enthusiastic hands, and, although many regarded the dissecting room as an important initiation for the young medical student, fortunately much of the detail needed for surgical practice is revised and extended later by observing and assisting at operations and during postgraduate training. Much more useful to general clinical practice is the increased teaching of living and radiological anatomy. In living anatomy, which is vital before trying to learn how to examine a patient, the surface markings of internal structures are learnt by using each other as models. This makes for a fun change from a stuffy lecture theatre as willing volunteers (and there are always one or two in every year) strip off to their smalls while some blushing colleague draws out the position of their liver and spleen with a felt tip marker pen.

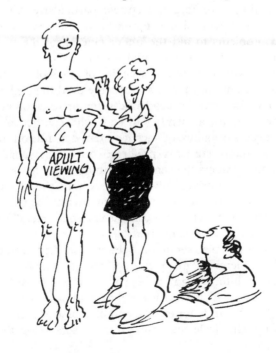

Similarly, with the technological advances in imaging parts of the body with x rays, ultrasound, computed tomography, magnetic resonance imaging, radionucleotide scans, and the like, and their subsequent use in both diagnosis and treatment, the need to have a basic understanding of anatomy through radiology has never been greater.

Practical sessions in other subjects, especially physiology and pharmacology, often involve students performing simple tests on each other under supervision. Memorable afternoons are recalled in the lab being tipped upside down on a special revolving table while someone checked my blood pressure or peddling on an exercise bike at 20 km/h for half an hour with a long air pipe in my mouth and a clip on my nose while my vital signs were recorded by highly entertained friends or recording the effect on the colour of my urine of eating three whole beetroots, feeling relieved not to be the one who had to test the effects of 20 fish oil capsules. As well as the performing of the experiments, the collation and analysis of the data and the researching and writing up of conclusions is seen as central to the exercise, and so students may find themselves being introduced to teaching in information technology, effective use of a library, statistics, critical reading of academic papers, and data handling and presentation skills.

The teaching of much of the early parts of the course is carried out by basic medical scientists, most of whom are not medically qualified but who are specialist researchers in their subject. Few have formal training in teaching but despite this the quality of the teaching is generally good and the widespread introduction of student evaluation of their teachers is pushing up standards even further. Small group tutorials play an important part in supplementing the more formal lectures, particularly when learning is centred around a problem solving approach, with students working through clinical based problems to aid the understanding of the system or topic being studied at that time. The tutorial system is also an important anchor point for students who find the self discipline of much of the learning harder than the spoon feeding they may have become used to at school.

Students may also have an academic tutor or director of studies or a personal tutor, or both, a member of staff who can act as a friend and adviser. The success or failure of such a system depends on the individuals concerned, and many students prefer to obtain personal advice from sympathetic staff members they encounter in their day to day course rather than seeking out a contrived adviser with whom they have little or no natural contact. In some schools, most notably in Oxbridge, the college based tutor system is much more established and generally plays a more important personal and academic part.

Links are sometimes also set up between new students and those in older years; these "link friends", "mentors", or "parents" can often be extremely useful sources of information on a whole range of issues from which textbooks to buy to which local general practitioner to register with and useful tips on how to study for exams, and of course numerous suggestions on how to spend what little spare time you can scrape together.

In every school there will be a senior member of staff, a sub-dean or director of medical education, who oversees the whole academic programme and can follow the progress of individuals and offer a guiding hand where needed.

As students progress other topics are added into the course. Most schools provide first aid training for their students, and a choice of special study modules (SSMs) are offered each year to encourage students to spend some time studying in breadth or depth an area which interests them and in which they can develop more knowledge and understanding. Early patient contact is encouraged; sometimes through schemes which link a junior student with a ward where small group teaching takes place or through projects or simply by gaining experience of the work of other staff, such as nurses, health visitors, physiotherapists, and occupational therapists; or time can be spent just talking to patients and relatives. Some schools begin a module in the first year which introduces aspects of clinical training, ideally in the setting of general practice, with the same doctor every week or two for one or two years. The supervised learning includes skills such as history taking and clinical examination or the interpretation of results of clinical investigations.

In the early part of some courses students may be introduced to a local family with whom they will remain in contact for the duration of their time as a student. Such attachment schemes, which are often organised by general practice departments, are designed to give students a realistic experience of the effects on people of events such as child birth, bereavement, financial hardship, or ill health from a perspective which few would otherwise encounter.

It is difficult to get the true feel of being in the early years of medical training from the rather dry description of the course, so let a student at that stage herself describe a typical week in her life on a new style problem based course.

A week on a problem-based learning course

Thursday

Yes, Thursday is the start of the week as far as we're concerned in Manchester. At least that's when we start each new case.

The idea behind problem-based learning (PBL) is that we use real clinical problems (or cases) as the main stimulus for our learning. Each week we have a new case to study; understanding the background to the problem itself and exploring aspects related to it. Nobody tells us what we "need" to know, we must decide for ourselves which information is important to learn and understand. At first, like everybody, I found it difficult to adjust to this new way of learning—I was used to the spoon fed process at school which helped me pass my A levels. I found it quite daunting and challenging to make up my own learning objectives and search out the information for myself. Once

I got used to it, however, it became a really enjoyable way to study medicine. I found myself actually wanting to spend time in the library or in hospital to find the answers to my questions. I quickly found out that there is no need to rote learn all the muscle attachments of the bones in the hand or every single anatomical feature of the femur. I learnt to discriminate between useless information and useful information—for example, how antidepressants work or the functions of the stomach.

In the past, medics on traditional courses spent their first two years trying to cram textbooks of information into their heads and usually hating every minute of it, desperately waiting for the clinical years. If you ask them how much information they retained after their preclinical exams were over they'll find it difficult to admit that they forgot nearly everything straightaway! By using the PBL method to learn medicine the information we learn now is more likely to be retained in the future, long after our exams when we're doctors on the wards. I discovered that it's a very satisfying way to learn medicine as I am constantly solving cases and applying my knowledge to real life situations. My motivation to learn is increased and because I actually want and like to learn I find it easier to understand and remember what I read about. It's one thing being able to learn facts and principles, it's quite another to apply them in real life. Problem based learning helps us to learn the skills necessary to do this—skills that we must learn to be good doctors.

In Manchester, the first two years are divided into four semesters. Each semester has a title—for example, Nutrition and Metabolism, Cardiorespiratory Fitness. This semester I am studying "Abilities and Disabilities", and it involves learning mainly about the brain, nervous system, muscles, and bones.

At 10 am I have a theatre event. This usually means going into the lecture theatre (hence the name!) to listen to a lecture, but sometimes we'll watch a video or take part in a clinical demonstration. The lectures are usually interactive too, and we're encouraged to ask questions or participate in discussion. The theatre event this morning introduced us to aspects of that week's case by giving us an overview of how the eye works. The patient in the case this week is followed from childhood (when she has a squint) through to old age (when her eyesight deteriorates, partly due to disease).

Afterwards I decided to go to the library for a couple of hours to read up before my first discussion group. Each week we study the case with our tutor group (consisting of about 12–15 students). We have 3 one hour meetings in the week to work through the case. This week, Mary is assigned the role of chairperson and Mike is scribe. The chairperson tries to keep the discussion on track (and keep us under control!) whereas the scribe has the job of writing the important points down during the session and typing them up. We rotate the two jobs each week so everyone has a chance. Each group has two tutors who are always present but usually do not take part in the discussion unless we ask them a specific question. One tutor is a basic medical scientist and the other is a clinician. The tutors are there to facilitate our discussion and will interrupt us only if we go off on a tangent. The clinician is also there as our main link to hospital and will invite us in to have small group teaching on the wards or will make it possible for us to come in pairs to shadow other doctors on shifts. In my first year I chose to spend a Saturday night in accident and emergency. Unfortunately (or fortunately!), it was not the

Casualty/ER scenario I expected, and two drunks and a regular were the only ones to come in during the entire 12 hour shift.

We usually read through the case in the first session, defining things we don't understand, using clues in the case to decide what we need to learn about, and dividing up the tasks between us. We form learning objectives based on the case itself, which means that we cover anatomy, physiology, biochemistry, pharmacology, psychology, etc, altogether instead of each subject being learned separately. I've found that this method of learning medicine, the "systems based" method, gives me a more complete picture and I'm able to connect up the anatomy, physiology, etc, of an organ better and remember how they are related to each other. It also means that we understand disease processes more thoroughly and that we're encouraged to look at the patient as a whole person within society not just as an illness.

Friday

I didn't have to be in for dissection until 11 am. We have two hours of dissection every week when we get hands on experience of the body and primarily discuss anatomy with a tutor in our tutor groups. Today we dissected the eye and the orbit of the brain of our cadaver. The first time I saw the cadaver was a moment I'll remember for ever, and I think dissection is one of the most interesting times of the week, the only thing I don't like is the smell! We also use this time to do living anatomy and look at *x* ray pictures and body scans.

Just had time to grab a sandwich from the coffee bar before the theatre event at 1 pm. This time it was a demonstration and video about how the eye detects colour, especially in the dark. It was really good fun, and we experimented with optical illusions.

Finished again at 3 pm and went to the library for an hour to learn more about colour vision but found it difficult to focus on the textbook at first since my eyes were still suffering from the optical illusions.

Weekend

I spent most of the weekend in the library, working on the case. Except for Saturday morning when I played in a mixed hockey match against Edinburgh medics. Medicine takes up a large part of my life but I always manage to find time to do other things.

Monday

Early start for computers at 9 am. We have two hours of computing class every week. We also learn about statistics during that time and how to carry out statistical procedures using the computer. I didn't do statistics at school but it's not a disadvantage since we are taken through things step by step. It's the same with computing so that even if you've never even switched one on before, it soon becomes possible to produce spreadsheets and data analyses.

At 11 am I have histology class. We also have two hours of histology a week. We work through the lesson in pairs with the help of tutors. Depending on the case, I sometimes find myself spending longer in the lab to make sure

I've seen everything that I'm supposed to see down the microscope. Although it can be fascinating this is not my favourite medical pastime.

That was it for the day and I was able to take my time over lunch. In the afternoon Lucy and I headed across to the Manchester Royal Infirmary. We eventually found the ophthalmology department and introduced ourselves to the nurses and met the consultant as arranged. We were able to see five patients during the three hours we were there, and it really opened my eyes to the treatments possible.

Tuesday

From 9–11 am we had lab work. This is the time when we learn how to carry out certain examinations or procedures, everything from blood pressure measurement to drug dilutions. This week we learnt how to examine the eye with an ophthalmoscope and carry out an eye test like you have done at the opticians. It was more complicated than it seemed, and it took me and my partner Toby the entire two hours to get through everything.

At noon we had our second discussion group. Lucy and I gave an account about what we'd seen on the ward, and Farid gave a presentation on how laser treatments work to improve eyesight. We discussed the case but realised there were still some aspects to it we didn't understand. Some people were assigned specific things to find out for tomorrow's session. We also agreed to go out for a group meal tomorrow night! We do this about twice each semester so we have some time to socialise together as a group.

At 3 pm we had another theatre event, this one was about eye surgery and the techniques they use—it was quite gruesome. At the end of the lecture we had a feedback session. Each semester we're asked to give our opinions on how the course is going and any improvements that we think should be made. We fill in lots of questionnaires about everything, from the books we use in the library to what we think of our tutors. The staff are really good and although PBL is now well established in its third year, they are still willing to make changes and genuinely listen to our problems. Students are actively involved in all faculty committees too.

We finished at 4 pm but I went to the computer lab to use one of the computer assisted learning (CAL) programmes. I like using them because they're more interactive than textbooks; they usually have quizzes so I can test myself at the end.

Wednesday

At 10 am we had our final discussion session about the case. It was quite a good session since we managed to tie up nearly all our loose ends and still had time to talk about the social issues that the case raised. Our clinical tutor gave us a clinical perspective on the case and told us a few of his experiences too.

The good thing about working in groups is that it helps us to develop our communication skills. We are always having to explain our theories and listen to each other, which means we get very good at talking about medicine. It is good preparation for us as future doctors as we'll have to do this constantly with patients. I've become very good at working in a team too—an invaluable skill to have as a doctor.

That evening we had a group night out and went for a curry. One of the best things about PBL is that you really get to know the people in your group very well because you work together as a team. You go through a lot together, and the groups are small enough to allow you to work closely with everyone during the semester.

I really enjoy studying medicine PBL style. It teaches you important and essential skills for being a doctor as well as being brilliant fun.

C-MB

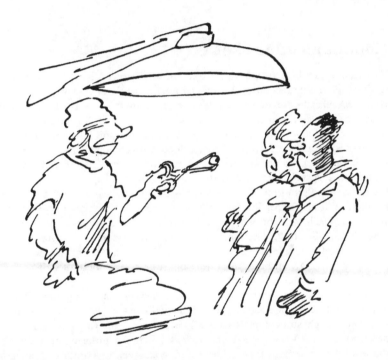

Communication skills

The teaching of communication skills to medical students has improved greatly across the board in recent years, largely in response to public demand. Patients want to know more about their condition and to have more involvement in the decisions, for instance about treatment options, which affect their lives. The skills needed to communicate well with patients are often not fully appreciated, and many, including well established doctors think it is something you either have or do not have.

While it is true that some doctors do have a natural flair for the right bedside manner and know instinctively when to hold a hand or when a moment of quiet reflection is appropriate, many of the skills can in fact be learnt quite easily. Such skills are not just about explaining procedures and breaking bad news but also about how and when to keep quiet and listen, to ask the right questions in the right way, drawing out the patient's story, which allows you to make an accurate diagnosis and formulate a suitable management plan, as well as earning trust and showing empathy. Much of this teaching is done in small groups and uses actors role playing patients with fellow students watching on television monitors. This type of training is also a compulsory part of postgraduate training in general practice, so the practice early on is time doubly well spent. Let a former student, now a medical senior house officer, describe her experiences of communication skills training.

Communication skills

You will be spending the rest of your prospective career talking to patients so it's nice to be able to do it well—indeed it's one of the major ways in which your medical skills are judged. To this end, the communication skills teaching is designed to give you a few pointers as to how to handle various patient scenarios so that you and the patient go away happy (and less liable to sue!).

There is a small group of students, a doctor, psychologist, and a TV/video at each session. You are in the room next door with an actor and a video camera to keep you company. Before it starts, all you can think of are your friends watching you on TV next door in this totally artificial situation and how stupid it all seems! But then the actor arrives playing your patient and you're away. They might be trying to tell you about their piles or of "trouble down below, Doctor". They may be a shy, retiring nun or the Marquis de Sade—anything is fair game. There are various scenarios and patients that the actors can play, and they are invariably superb. You forget it's all a sham and that your friends are next door watching you on TV.

A particular favourite that you are asked to do is explain to a patient (actor) a special test he or she needs to have done and what it will be like for him or her. The old chestnut is endoscopy. This usually leads to some wonderful descriptions of TV cameras being forced down the unfortunate patient's throat which, judging by their aghast expressions, seems to conjure up images of the cameraman, floor manager, and producer going down to have a look, too! The most difficult to explain are tests involving the injection of a harmless radioactive isotope. On at least one occasion the patient left the room convinced his hair would fall out and his skin peel and blister in a most Chernobyl-esque manner!

After the consultation you go back next door and receive comments from those watching. Emphasis is put on your good points as well as your goofs, so it boosts your confidence (that's half the trick in good communication) for dealing with real patients, as well as raising your awareness of the possible pitfalls. Invaluable skills are learnt, which past students—now doctors—say they are still using on the wards now.

LJ

Intercalated honours degrees

An increasing number of students are choosing to spend an extra year studying for an honours degree during the medical course. This is usually a Bachelor of Science (BSc) or Bachelor of Medical Science (BMedSci) and can usually be taken from the end of the second year to the beginning of the final year, depending on the design of the course and the exact nature of the subject being studied. These degrees can either have a more basic science emphasis—for example, extending study from a SSM in neurosciences or neonatal physiology—or if it is taken later in the course some schools offer clinical science related degrees. This extra year of study is often the only opportunity an undergraduate has to experience front line scientific research; besides the subject knowledge gained, it is a unique chance to develop skills in research and laboratory techniques, and writing scientific papers. Occasionally there are opportunities for a much broader range of study encompassing humanities such as history of medicine or modern languages. There are numerous grants and scholarships available from schools and research funds to assist with the expense of this additional year to cover living expenses if not tuition fees. Despite the extra expense the number of students seeing the advantages of making the sacrifices needed to take up this valuable opportunity is continuing to grow.

There are several notable exceptions to the general design of the intercalated degrees being outlined here. At St Andrew's University the student takes a three year (or four if an honours degree) preclinical course leading to a BSc in Medical Sciences and then usually transfers to clinical studies at Manchester University. At both Imperial College School of Medicine and the Royal Free and University College London School of Medicine a six year course includes a modular BSc (Hons) as well as the MB BS. At Nottingham University, all students on the five year course are awarded a BMedSci if they successfully complete the first three years, which includes research based project work.

The other main exceptions are the courses at Oxford and Cambridge, whose first three years lead to a Bachelor of Arts degree, in Medical Sciences at Cambridge and Physiological Sciences at Oxford.

Occasionally a student who has a particular research interest continues the BSc break in their medical course to complete a further three years of advanced research leading to the award of Doctor of Philosophy (PhD). Some medical schools such as Cambridge and University College, London, offer selected students a combined MB/PhD which is shorter than taking the two degrees separately.

Assessment

The variety and complexity of the courses offered by different medical schools are reflected in the numerous types of assessment used to check the progress of each student's learning. Attendance is not usually checked, but a student who is thought to be missing large amounts of the course should expect to be questioned by tutors and the senior tutor to discover whether there are any major problems with which the school may be able to help. Like most university courses the obligation to attend is the responsibility of the student, and it is salutary to note that poor course attendance, for whatever reason, corresponds highly with failing the early phases of the course.

Most schools use a mixture of continuous assessment of course work and major examinations at the end of terms or years, though the balance varies greatly. There are pros and cons of both systems, with students at schools where exams play a larger part wishing that more credit were given to good work throughout the year rather than everything resting on their performance on one particular day. Students who undergo more continuous assessment, however, complain about the stresses and strains of frequent tests and projects, so it seems to be a case of "swings and roundabouts".

Around 5% of students fail to complete the course, most of these leaving at the end of the first year. This is most commonly due to a waning of motivation, the realisation of a wrong career choice, or, unfortunately, because of misjudgments of the amount of work necessary and a failure to organise their time effectively or because of the diversions of personal entanglements. A few fail their second or third year assessments, but students surviving this far have generally worked out what is required of them to qualify.

There is often a chance to resit examinations or resubmit unsatisfactory course work, but this is not to be recommended as it leads to extra work often at times when friends are away on vacations, sunning themselves on faraway beaches or earning much needed cash in holiday jobs. In exceptional circumstances, such as illness or bereavement, students may be allowed to resit a whole year, but this often has financial implications which may preclude some people. In any event, students who are experiencing difficulties are encouraged to discuss the problems with their tutor or another member of staff sooner rather than later.

Working hard, playing hard

On my first day at medical school the then president of the Royal College of Radiologists, Dr Oscar Craig, told the assembled mass of eager freshers, "this is the greatest day of your life". He continued, "Does it take great brains to become a doctor? I hate to disappoint you, but I don't think it does, you know. Does it take hard work and determination? ... Like nothing else!"

Students who have gained a place at medical school have not only proved themselves bright enough to cope with the academic rigours of the course but have also usually shown exceptional interest or achievement in some other area or activity, often an activity requiring teamwork. It is usual then for medical schools to be hives of activity on the social scene, where clubs and societies abound providing sports fixtures, training sessions, plays and concerts, balls and discos, talks on this and that, and trips to here and there, all of which can lead to a wonderfully full life.

While the object of going to medical school is ultimately to train as a doctor, most students take full advantage of the chance to pursue their hobbies or try new ones, meet new friends, do new things, and generally do all the "growing up and finding yourself" things that students are supposed to do. The secret in all this is the fine balancing act between work and play. Each year a few potentially good doctors forget the real reason for their being at medical school, fail their exams, and have to leave their friends and all that social life behind, not to mention having to find a new career. It is an unpleasant feeling seeing a good friend and colleague being asked to leave, so a great effort is made to encourage students to find the right balance so that medical schools train doctors who are both skilled at their job and also interesting and talented in other things; something they will cherish in later life.

REMEMBER

- Being a medical student, like any university student, is a complete change from being at school—you will have endless opportunities available to you but you will need to realise them for yourself.

- There is generally much less "spoon feeding" and more self-directed learning, requiring self-motivation, determination and discipline, which some students find difficult at first.

- All medical courses now provide early clinical insights and problem solving in addition to teaching the scientific and ethical basis of medicine.

- Courses range from the recognisably traditional at Oxford, Cambridge, and St Andrew's to substantially more integrated, problem-based approaches such as at Liverpool and Manchester.

- Several universities have introduced shorter (four year) courses for graduate students.

- A few universities award a science degree as an integral part of the medical course; most universities award a BSc or BMedSci degree for an optional, additional (intercalated) year.

- Assessment in the early years is by a variable mixture of continuous assessments and end of year exams.

- Achieving the right balance between work and play can be a challenge for some new medical students, but most succeed.

- About 5% of students overall fail to complete the course, most in the first two years and they normally find fulfilling careers outside medicine.

8. Medical school: the later years

As the medical student progresses through into their third year and beyond, increasing amounts of time are spent in the various clinical teaching settings and less in the classroom. The white coat is donned, and the shiny new stethoscope is placed ostentatiously in the pocket, usually alongside numerous pocket-sized textbooks, pens, notepads, and sweet wrappers. Most students by now have some experience of listening and talking to patients and of the hospital wards. The sight of the ill patient in a bed does not come as the awful surprise it did to generations of medical students who spent their first two years cocooned in the medical school.

The style of teaching changes emphasis, becoming more of an apprenticeship but retaining the academic backup of lectures, seminars, and particularly tutorials. More of the course is taught by clinical staff: consultants, general practitioners, and junior doctors, often in small groups at the bedside, on dedicated teaching rounds or in tutorials, in the operating theatre, in the outpatient clinic, or general practice surgery. Teaching also takes place at clinical meetings or Grand Rounds and the firm's regular radiology meeting (when the week's x ray pictures and scans are reviewed and discussed with a radiologist) and histopathology meeting (when the results of tissue biopsies and postmortem examinations are discussed). Some students find the change in the style of teaching frustrating as much time seems to be wasted hanging around waiting for teaching that never seems to happen. The registrar or consultant who is due to be teaching is often delayed in theatre with a difficult case or still has a queue of patients waiting in the outpatient clinic. Many of these doctors are fitting in their teaching commitments around an already punishing clinical workload, and so often a combination of better organisation by the schools and some initiative in self directed learning from the students is all that is needed to extract the value from such a valuable educational source.

It may well be that with so much to learn, insufficient attention is given to the formation of attitudes. It is said that medical students have more appropriate attitudes to both patients and to others with whom they share care when they enter medical school than when they qualify as doctors. There may be more than a grain of truth in this. In the Bristol report,

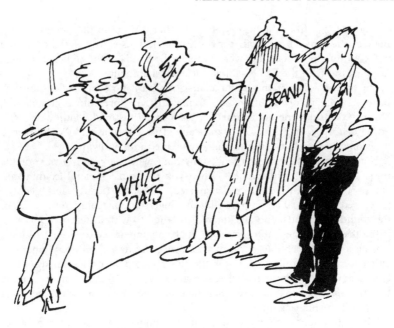

Professor Sir Ian Kennedy expressed the view that "the education and training of all healthcare professionals should be imbued with the idea of partnership ... (with) ... the patient ... whereby the patient and the professional meet as equals". As far as mutual respect in teamwork is concerned, opportunities for learning together (multidisciplinary learning), both in the undergraduate and postgraduate years, are not fully exploited.

Much can be learned from reasonable complaints. A patient who had complained about the attitude of his surgeon was interviewed by another surgeon as part of a formal investigation into the complaint. The patient was pleased to find that the investigating surgeon was a complete contrast— "conversational, sympathetic, and informative; wide ranging and encouraged questions (with) a very human approach which inspired trust." As the complainant explained, the matter need never have reached the stage of formal complaint: all he had been seeking was "a small acceptance (from the first surgeon) that some of the procedures are inadequate and will be revised". Arrogance is something that students need to lose early in their training, if they have the misfortune to be afflicted by it; patients can do without it.

First patients

Stepping tentatively on to the ward for the first time, resplendent in my new white coat, I felt that the long awaited moment had arrived. "Clerking" involves taking a history from and examining the patient. We had been told that this process, which has been handed down from doctor to medical student for countless generations, enables the doctor to make 95% of the diagnosis (75% from the history and a further 20% from the examination—the last 5% comes from further investigations). This is why clerking has and will continue to be such a powerful tool in the hands of the clinician, though not necessarily in the hands of a junior clinical student.

On the first day of the junior course we learn how to take a thorough history. This involves an overall framework of "presenting complaint", "history of presenting complaint", "past medical history", "family history", "drug history", "social history", and "any other information". With practice it becomes possible to tailor the history taking to the individual.

Next comes the examination, something which opens up a veritable minefield for the inexperienced. When you perform a general examination every body system has to be inspected, palpated (lightly and deeply), percussed (examined by tapping with the fingers and listening to the pitch of the sound produced), and auscultated (listened to with a stethoscope). This is the theory but inevitably, either through incompetence or sheer bad luck, it is almost impossible to perform a perfect examination on every patient—either some of the pulses are not felt or the enlarged liver does not seem that enlarged; whatever the sign of disease that causes such frustration by escaping the student, you can guarantee that the senior house officer will come along and find it within seconds!

The introduction to basic surgical techniques was one of the better activities organised for us during the junior clinical course. Armed with scalpels, sutures, forceps, and pigs trotters the surgeons demonstrated the basic principles of stitching wounds and then let us loose on our own practice limbs. This was an excellent afternoon for the students, not least because it gave us the opportunity to do something incredibly practical that most of us had never done before. Having mastered (?) the mattress stitch, we moved on to the more cosmetically friendly subcuticular stitch, and I am sure we greatly impressed our surgical superiors with our manual dexterity!

The afternoon concluded with teaching us how to draw up and mix drugs with a syringe and how to inject them subcutaneously and intramuscularly (the intramuscular route was cleverly improvised with an orange).

My first firm was a series of firsts. First clerking of a patient—nerve racking as the whole scenario is new. I felt ill equipped and slightly obtrusive as I clumsily searched, questioned, and of course palpated and percussed my patient. The sense of relief as I parted the curtains and left the cubicle, history complete, was overwhelming.

First ward round—how I regretted not learning my anatomy better as in the words of our senior registrar I displayed "chasms of ignorance", only managing to redeem myself by the narrowest of margins.

First surgical operation—it was a real privilege to clerk a patient, then later watch and even assist in the operation and later still revisit the patient on the ward. Theatre also provided a superb way to learn by watching but also by the excellent active teaching of the surgeons.

First freedom—for the first time since entering medical school I was expected to decide for myself what to go to, what to learn, what to read, and to think more laterally and broadly than ever before.

First encounter with real patients with lives we are able to be part of for some small time—call us naive and overenthusiastic and we would agree. We are sure that some of the novelty will wear off after nights on take and unpleasant patients. Call us idealistic and we would agree and pray that it may be a comment levelled at us not just now as we experience our "firsts" but on until we experience our very "lasts". When idealism dies it is not replaced by realism but by cynicism and long may we be idealistic realists.

AH, SC

Meanwhile, at another medical school, another student was seeing a similar experience through somewhat different eyes.

First clinical "firm"

The first day as a clinical student is a little like the first time you have sex. There is a lot of anxiety and excitement for what often ends up as a disappointing and humiliating experience. At last an escape from lecture halls and seminar rooms; an end to being force fed mind numbing facts such as the course of the left recurrent laryngeal nerve or the intricacies of gluconeogenesis. I had a crisp white coat and smart matching shirt and tie. The finishing touch being a stethoscope slung casually around my neck. I had arrived, I looked fantastic, and I was IT.

I was attached to a firm run by a consultant whose fearsome reputation was unrivalled in the region. She had a moustache that Stalin would have been proud of and a personality to match. My fellow students were a real mixed bag; two rugby lads, two sloanes, a girly swot, a computer geek, and a goth! Most medical students wear a common uniform; boys in light blue shirts, stripy ties (preferably rugby ties), chinos (regulation length one inch too short), and either shiny, pointy shoes or those brown deck shoe things. Girls tend to opt for simple blouses with pretty necklines and floaty, flowery, shapeless skirts ... invariably sensible and never fashionable.

Every aspect of being a clinical student combines in an attempt both to educate you and to expose you to the realities of being a junior doctor. The time is split between seeing patients on the wards, teaching sessions, sitting in clinics, and assisting in operating theatres. The day usually begins with a ward round. Medicine is like a huge machine; everyone has an allocated role; everyone is an essential moving part. The system works well if we all know our place and act according to our roles. The ward round reflects this system and demonstrates the hierarchy and tradition that exists in medicine. The consultant is the boss. His (or less commonly her) role is twofold. Firstly, to impart knowledge to the more junior members of the team (that is, everyone) in the form of witty and wise anecdotes and, secondly, to use derision, disapproval or old-fashioned humiliation on his or her juniors lest they forget their places.

Next in line are the registrars who are occasionally allowed to adopt the role of the consultant if he or she is otherwise engaged at the golf course/race course/Harley Street. Very rarely registrars are allowed to know something the consultant doesn't. There are strict limitations on what this information can be, but it generally involves very obscure areas of research that will never

75

make it into the textbooks anyway! The senior house officers and house officers ensure the smooth running of the firm; taking notes, making lists, organising tests, and collecting results. They are also objects for ritual humiliation (that is, teaching) when the students are not around. Your role as a student is not difficult; laugh at the consultant's jokes, help out when needed, learn lots, and make great tea.

I was strangely reassured to find that ward rounds conformed to my preconceived idea of an all powerful consultant sweeping down the ward with an entourage of doctors and students following in order of decreasing seniority. Each student is allocated their own patients. On this particular day, my luck is in; the procession stops at the bedside of a young asthmatic man with a chest infection. He is not my patient. The student concerned steps forward, a little flushed and sweaty, but none the less does a good job of presenting her case and answers well under interrogation from the consultant. Her triumph, however, is short lived. It is revealed that she has not looked in the patient's sputum pot for three days. This is just short of a hanging offence on a respiratory firm!

There are a number of skills that make life as a medical student more tolerable. Most of these involve creating the impression that you know more than you actually do. This means avoiding answering questions about which you know nothing (which at the beginning is most things). Consider the ritual of bedside teaching. I made it my mission to avoid speaking to or touching the patients at all costs. Avoiding eye contact is a guaranteed way to be asked a question! All patients are examined from the right hand side, therefore initially it is advisable to stand on the left hand side of the patient. One needs to judge the time accurately, however, when the clinician will try to be cunning and ask the student standing the *furthest away* from the patient. The skilled student will anticipate this moment and, at the appropriate time, enthusiastically stands on the right of the patient, hence double bluffing the clinician. When successful this manoeuvre is poetry in motion.

After clinic I went to the casualty department as it was my turn to shadow the house officer on call. This turns out to be highly enjoyable; seeing real patients with real diseases and being involved in the process of sorting them out without the responsibility of having to *know* things or make decisions. In the space of a few hours we see two old ladies with chest infections, a man with heart failure, two paracetamol overdoses, and a heart attack. A moment's peace some four or five hours later is shattered by a series of piercing bleeps and a crackling disjointed voice proclaims from the house officer's pocket that there has been a cardiac arrest on one of the wards. The dreaded crash bleep: we get up, and we run. We arrive on the ward, and very quickly there is a small crowd of doctors and nurses around the bed of the old man we had admitted earlier with a heart attack. I stand back feeling more than a little useless. Intrigued and a little appalled, I watch as the registrar gives instructions to insert lines and tubes and to administer drugs and electric shocks. After about 20 minutes everything stops; a stillness replaces the activity and the old gentleman is left to rest in peace. I feel upset and shocked, but to everyone else it's just part of the job.

The clinical years are the first real opportunity to manage your own time. It is important to do so sensibly. The system is open to abuse and many a cunning student manages to do the minimum amount of work in the shortest period of time. There will be things you love about being a student and things you'll hate. I personally would avoid operating theatres like the plague. There is nothing pleasant about standing around in green pyjamas, a paper shower cap, and fetid, communal shoes in which most decent people would not even grow mushrooms, never mind put their feet. The student in theatre is meant to *retract*. This involves pulling very hard on metal implements (which are usually inserted in a stranger's abdomen) in directions that your body was not designed to go. This causes pain, stiffness, and eventually loss of sensation in the hands, the likes of which have never been felt before outside a Siberian salt mine.

It is important to learn the things you need to get through the exams, but there are a lot of other valuable lessons to learn. One day you will be a house officer and your social life and sanity will be seriously compromised ... so don't waste the time you have now. Medicine *is* great, with something to appeal to everyone. It's a little like a pomegranate: you will hopefully find it satisfying and worth while in the end, but it can be challenging and infuriating going through the process!

MB

Self directed learning plays an ever increasing part as time goes on through the course and as you will be repeatedly reminded "every patient is a learning opportunity". There are always patients to be clerked and examined. This may be in the holistic mould of learning about the person, their condition, and the whole experience of their illness or learning the clinical features and management of the diseases relating to the specialty you are currently studying. Students nearing their clinical finals adopt a rather more focused approach: racing around the wards examining "the massive liver in bed 4", "the wheezy chest in bed 9", and the "rather embarrassing rash in the sideward", grabbing a quick coffee while firing questions at each other about the causes of finger clubbing and the side effects of amiodarone, then fitting in a couple of children and a mad person before lunch.

Keen students who spend more time on the wards seeing patients and learning about conditions for themselves often benefit from impromptu, informal teaching from junior doctors who can teach during the course of completing their ward work. Following a junior doctor on call is very valuable experience and is often the best way to see a general mix of cases. Students need to be around when things happen if they are not only to learn but to experience the excitement and satisfaction of clinical medicine. A group of students once reported on their experience in these words:

Our teaching was really, really good from house officers right through to consultants. So much time and effort was put in for us at all hours of the night and day, so much so that some of us learnt some important skills like how to read ECGs in the early hours of the morning on take in the hospital.

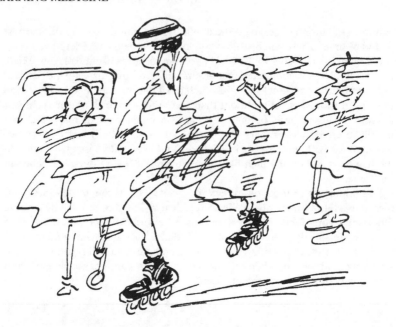

Spending an evening with the registrar in the accident and emergency department on the front line, seeing patients brought in by ambulance or referred by local general practitioners, is far more interesting for most students than standing at the back of an operating theatre, craning your neck, and still not being able to see what the surgeon is doing and getting flustered when you are shouted at for getting in the way or because you have momentarily forgotten the anatomical borders of Hasselback's triangle.

A night in casualty

I remember my first night in casualty as a medical student as one of the most exciting times of my whole medical training. My placement in what is properly called accident and emergency medicine was relatively early in my time at medical school so, although I felt that my knowledge was minimal, my enthusiasm levels had never been higher; how many other students would be excited at the prospect of spending all of Friday night doing college work? The department resembled Piccadilly Circus, in all senses, especially noise and smell. There was a constant flow of people milling here and rushing there, lying on trolleys, sitting on floors, banging on the wall, singing in the toilet, crying in the corner, or sleeping in the waiting room; men, women, children, patients, relatives, doctors, nurses, porters, receptionists, radiographers, a couple of burly policemen and a rather conspicuous and obvious plain clothed detective, and to cap it all two nuns looking for a missing mother superior.

As well as the large number of walking wounded, an increasing proportion of whom as the night wore on and the pubs closed became staggering wounded, there were a couple of cases which I think I will never forget as they showed me medicine in all its glory. A lovely lady in her 80s was brought in by ambulance, acutely short of breath and looking extremely distressed and scared. She had heart failure and her lungs were filling up with fluid as her heart could no longer pump effectively. Within minutes the junior doctor I was following around had put in a drip and was giving her some drugs which I had learnt about only a few weeks before in a tutorial. As I stood by her bed filling in the blood forms trying to help out a bit, she started to get her breath back and soon was able to talk to me. Within an hour she had managed to tell me her whole life story, including her several boyfriends during the war, the relevance of which to her medical history I still find hard to grasp, but she insisted it was important. About 2 am a young man of my age was rushed in from a road traffic accident, having been knocked off his motorcycle at high speed. He was unconscious and had several broken bones. Seemingly out of nowhere an enormous group of doctors and nurses appeared in the resuscitation room and pounced on the man, but with awe inspiring calm and organisation; it really was like watching an episode of *Casualty*, except that on TV you get a better view than you do when you are right at the back of a group of frantically busy people and you are trying not to get in the way. By 3.30 am everything had quietened down somewhat, though the waiting area was still half full. The motorcyclist was in theatre having one of his fractures screwed together, and the sweet old lady with an interesting history was apparently soundly asleep on a ward, one of the lucky few not having to stay on a trolley in casualty. I wandered off to bed exhausted and exhilarated; the doctors and nurses carried on seeing patients. How, I wondered, will I ever know what to do and be able to treat people as well as they did, and, more worrying, how will I be able to stay awake that long?

GR

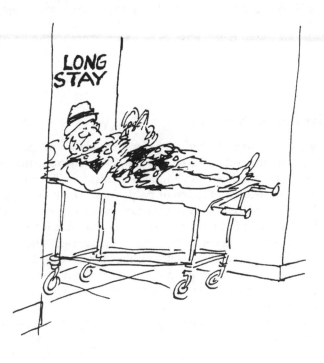

One of the most valuable experiences towards the end of training, which most schools encourage, is a period of several weeks shadowing a junior doctor. This usually occurs in medicine, surgery, or obstetrics and may take place in a general hospital away from the medical school. This allows only one or two students to be placed in each location, maximising their exposure to patients and teaching, and giving the opportunity for close supervision as clinical skills such as bladder catheterisation or intravenous cannulation are practised.

First delivery

I was woken up by the sound of my bleep. It was barely 4 am, and I had been asleep for less than two hours. By the time I had wearily put on my shoes and rushed to her cubicle, she had already begun to push. Jane, the midwife, decided that there was not time for me to put on a gown, so I just put on the gloves. The mother to be began to scream as the contractions became stronger and with each push the baby descended further. I placed my left hand on the head as the crown appeared to stop it rushing out too quickly, while supporting the mother with my right. I could almost feel my heart thumping against my chest. Any remaining signs of tiredness had now completely disappeared in all the excitement. Here I was minutes away from helping to bring a new life into the world.

It all went so quickly after that. First the baby's head appeared, and I pulled it down gently to release the anterior shoulder. The rest appeared to come out all by itself. It was 4.36 am precisely, and a big baby boy was born. The mother cried with joy as I placed him on her tummy. It's an amazing feeling. The family wouldn't let me go until they had taken a photograph of me holding him in my arms. By the time I had helped the midwife clear the mess and made sure all was well, it was way past 5 am. Time to get some sleep.

FI

The clinical subjects

The major subjects to be learnt are general medicine and general surgery, and these are often studied in several blocks throughout the later years. Increasingly, the emphasis is on core clinical skills rather than an encyclopaedic knowledge of different disciplines. The boundaries between "subjects" are blurred and they are learned in a more integrated way and examined in integrated clinical exams. If they are not integrated, and as medicine and surgery become ever more specialised, the best general experience is often achieved by rotating through several firms covering a range of subjects as well as being around when the firm is "on take" (the team responsible for general admissions on that day). An eight week medical attachment may involve a fortnight each of chest medicine, infectious diseases, endocrinology, and cardiology. A similar rotation in

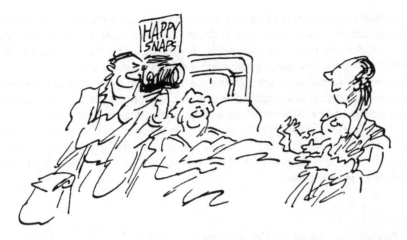

surgery could include gastrointestinal surgery, vascular surgery, urology, and orthopaedics.

Generally, students are split into small groups and allocated to a particular firm in the relevant specialty. The firm is the working unit of hospital medicine and usually comprises a consultant or professor, one or two specialist registrars (who qualified several years before and are in training for that specialty), a senior house officer (who is usually a couple of years out of medical school and may be wanting to follow that specialty or may be in training for general practice or may just be drifting waiting for inspiration), and a house officer (who is newly qualified and will try and whisper the answers to the boss's questions to you, which is generally why you will get them wrong).

The patients in hospital (inpatients) under the care of that team also provide the teaching subjects for the students and are shared out between the students, who are expected to talk to their patients and examine them before being taught on ward rounds or teaching sessions by the senior members of the team. In the past much of this teaching was in the form of humiliation; ritualistic grillings of students in front of patient and colleagues alike, in the style of Richard Gordon's character Sir Lancelot Spratt and his blustering, "You boy! What's the bleeding time. Speak up. Speak up". While the occasional medical dinosaur can still be found eating a brace of medical students for lunch, it is no longer acceptable today and is much less likely to occur. The student who has taken the effort to prepare for such teaching can gain enormous benefit from seeing a condition he or she has previously only read about being illustrated in flesh and blood, making far easier the committing to memory of facts and figures as they suddenly take on real meaning and significance.

The use of community-based services as resources for learning is growing in all schools, some at a faster rate than others. For example, Bristol now has a series of clinical academies across the West Country in Bath, Swindon, and Taunton for instance, where students spend several months at a time on attachment to various teaching firms. As more care passes from hospital to community, such as in mental illness or child health, and as hospital stays tend to be much shorter, such as after having a baby or having day surgery, students are having to go to where the patients are.

General practitioners are playing an increasing part in undergraduate teaching of clinical skills, such as examination of body systems, in addition to their traditional role of teaching consultation skills and health promotion. Insight can also be gained into a broader spectrum of disease and social problems than is apparent in hospitals, learning to deal appropriately with minor everyday illnesses or major personal upheavals that affect people's lives.

A day in general practice

My practice starts the day with a team meeting. A coffee fix gives everyone time to label the important events of the next few days. The builders are in, so all hearts will have a continuous murmur today; a new software package will be demonstrated to allow current problems to be highlighted while listing previous diagnoses, but will it really help? Instantly I am involved, my opinion sought in a warm welcome to the group. I ask what book I should read to learn about general practice and am told *Middlemarch* by George Eliot. Six months later, having read the book, I am still thinking about what was meant by that answer. In return, they ask me what skills a doctor should have in general practice. Everyone joins in, and the discussion leads us into seeing the patients.

Today I see the patients on my own first. I receive more trust and responsibility from these doctors in a week than in a year at the hospital. Presenting the complaint and my thoughts to the GP is excellent practice at developing a "problem-oriented approach". I am daunted by the impossibility of knowing the person and their history in 10 minutes, and hospital clerkings are little preparation. The long relationship between GP and patient is such a privilege and opportunity for appropriate intervention relevant to the patient's needs and wishes.

I think through the messages I learnt from watching myself on video being "consulted" by actors back at the St Mary's department of general practice. The skills are those of good listening, while considering the possible background to the presenting problem—the family problems, alcoholism—and the needs, articulated or unspoken, for caring, a further specialist opinion, or a prescription. I remember the advice that a holistic viewpoint and the availability of complementary therapies can obviate the need for drugs as psychological props for either doctor or patient.

Mr A has low back pain and was given short shrift by the orthopaedic consultant for not having sciatica that would be worth operating on, entirely ignoring his pain. We talk about his weight, posture, and stress at work and re-emphasise his need for exercises and a good chair, which seems more appropriate. Ms B comes in with severe abdominal pain and iliac fossa pain and rebound tenderness. My excitement at a possible hospital referral dies down as the doctor reassures both of us that this is constipation. The case mix is so different in a teaching hospital; a sense of proportion is vital and can come only with experience. Mr C was found to be hypertensive opportunistically at a previous visit, and the nurse has confirmed this subsequently. We discuss what this implies for his future health and treatment, and the doctor and I talk afterwards about current concepts in the management of blood pressure from both personal care and population health perspectives. Every person is different and requires integrating an understanding of the possible pathologies with what is realistic in their life. Without time or fast investigations nearly every diagnosis may be provisional; "come back tomorrow" is not a cop-out but good management.

In the corridor we have a "kerbside" case conference about what to do with Ms X. She has many problems, and all the partners have been to visit her at one time or other. The latest news is not good, and, although she has heart failure, it is her mobility and risk of hip fracture that we worry about. We visit her before lunch, assess her cardiovascular and neurological status, and find out how well the carers are coping. It may be that improving the lighting will counter her drowsiness and prevent a disastrous fall.

Over lunch we discuss strategies and priorities in looking after someone with diabetes and the implications for general practitioners of the new NHS changes. The balance has swung away from clinical freedom; doctors have lost much control over their time and decisions but to quite an extent are being forced to do what they would have liked to do anyway, namely more work on prevention and health promotion. Computerisation has been unavoidable but as yet wastes far more time than it saves. There is great potential for clear presentation of patient information and for networking outcomes between patients and practices for audit and research. I sit in quietly as another partner runs a yoga class in her lunchbreak and feel greatly refreshed for the afternoon.

Later on, I join the local community psychiatric nurse. One of the people we visit has panic attacks when she goes outside. The nurse has given her mental exercises to do at home and a routine to use when she feels the panic attack developing. We take her out for a walk calmly and get along without her anxiety becoming panic, which encourages her greatly. Another woman has gradually become more depressed since her husband died, and the nurse is delighted that she has a chance to intervene with counselling and cognitive therapy before a doctor (not from my practice!) has filled her full of tricyclic antidepressants. A third has Alzheimer's disease, and the issue is whether she will leave the frying pan on and burn the house down while her son is out at work.

Back at the practice I get on my bike to go home, overwhelmed by the breadth of insight needed in this work. The loneliness in the consulting room is more than compensated by the warmth of genuine teamwork and equal exchange of views and approaches. Humanity and pathophysiology do mix after all.

TA

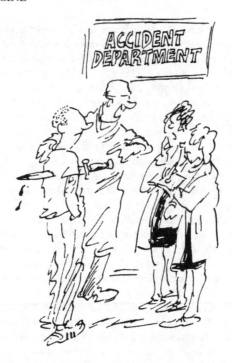

The major clinical subjects in addition to medicine and surgery are also taught in a similar fashion: obstetrics (the care of pregnant women) and gynaecology (the specialty devoted to diseases confined to women); paediatrics (child health); and psychiatry (the care of patients with mental illness).

Other specialties occupy a smaller part of the students' time, and only a general understanding is required as detailed knowledge is beyond the scope of basic general medical training. These include neurology (disorders of the motor and sensory function of the brain, spinal cord, and peripheral nerves); rheumatology (medical disorders of joints such as arthritis); genitourinary medicine (sexually transmitted diseases which may involve the study and care of HIV and AIDS); dermatology (skin diseases); ophthalmology (eye diseases); ear, nose, and throat surgery; and anaesthetics, which also covers pain management.

An attachment in the accident and emergency department is one of the most popular parts of the course for most students. The glamorous image portrayed by TV series is never all it is cracked up to be, but the excitement level is generally high, especially when there is the chance to be a useful pair of hands, suturing a laceration, helping the nurse put a plaster cast on the broken arm of a wriggling 5 year old, or providing chest compressions during a resuscitation.

At some stage in the later years a more detailed approach to pathology is required, and this may take the form of a block of lectures, tutorials, and practicals or may be covered throughout the later years alongside the

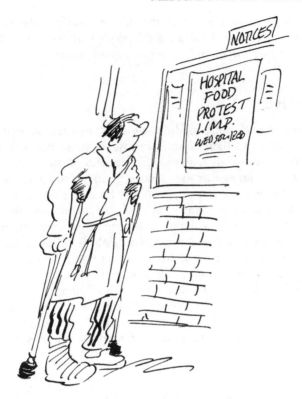

relevant clinical attachments. The subjects studied under the heading of pathology are chemical pathology (the biochemical basis of diseases); histopathology (the macro and microscopic structure of diseased tissues); haematology (the diseases affecting blood and bone marrow); microbiology (combining the study of bacteria, viruses, and other infectious organisms); and immunology (the role of the immune system in disease). Without a knowledge of these disease processes it is difficult to understand clinical signs and symptoms and to interpret the results of laboratory tests which play a crucial part in diagnosis and management of patients.

Other topics are fitted in as the course progresses including clinical pharmacology and therapeutics (the prescribing of drugs to treat illness), palliative medicine (the care of the dying), medical law and ethics, more advanced communication skills such as breaking bad news and bereavement counselling, and sometimes personal care (how to look after yourself with all the physical and emotional stresses and strains of being a doctor) and basic management skills. An increasing number of medical schools also give students a general introduction to complementary and alternative medicine, so that as doctors they may have at least some insight into their patients' choices and also consider whether some aspects, such as acupuncture, might become a useful adjunct to their own practice. The aim of the later years is to build on the basic knowledge and skills learnt in the early years and to add to that the necessary attitudes and skills in decision making, coping with uncertainty, and dealing effectively with patients, relatives, and colleagues that patients should expect of a good doctor.

The elective

As well as the special study modules which allow each student choices in the precise content of their course, and the opportunity to learn how to study in greater depth, all schools set time aside in the later years of the course for what is known as the elective period. This is usually between 6 and 12 weeks long and is an opportunity for a student to undertake any medically related study at home or abroad. Most students take the chance to travel and see medicine being practised in a very different setting whether in a trauma unit in down town Washington DC, the Australian Flying Doctor Service, or a children's immunisation clinic in a canoe in Sarawak. Some students carry out research while on elective or gain experience of a subject to which they have only limited exposure in their undergraduate course such as learning difficulties or tropical diseases. The *British Medical Journal* offers a different sort of opportunity through the Clegg scholarship for electives working in medical journalism.

A day on elective

Breakfast is pawpaw and aromatic coffee with sacred ibis calling as they fly along the Indian ocean shore. The day starts with the ward round. Eighty kids are packed two or three to a bed. They variously smile or cry, run around fighting or lie listlessly, bellies bulging with kwashiorkor or skin, eyes, and hope flaccid with dehydration. I stride into the measles side ward, a tiny room with three cots now packed with 10 mothers and babies in various stages of spottiness.

Admitting a child with measles is easy. The repertoire of a 1 year old is limited to vomiting, diarrhoea, fever, cough, and breathlessness, and with measles all are present in abundance. Red eyes, throat, and eardrums complete the picture examined carefully on the mother's knee (not my own after it was drenched on day one), and the vague but, with experience, characteristic graininess that will pass for a rash on black skin the next day is hardly needed. The mothers know it to be measles anyway. This is not my benign childhood discomfort of measles. Many of them will die of bronchopneumonia (ampicillin is probably just to keep the doctors happy, but we watch carefully for signs of staphylococci) or of dehydration, which has become my personal crusade. My five minute lecture in broken Swahili attempts to persuade the mother to take on the responsibility of forcing in rehydration fluid tirelessly. So my round of the measles ward is basically to take the temperature and respiratory rate and get a general feeling for each child's health. The sick ones get a closer look that always comes down to not enough water, and so, to the general amusement of all, I'm back on my hobby horse for a bit more negotiating about why the child won't drink or is not getting enough.

Talking about fluids and measles has been fascinating. Discussions in small groups, wandering round the rickety shacks both in town and out in the surrounding forest, stumble on in Swahili or are translated from Giriama by the wonderful local fieldworker who introduces me. Drunken men lolling in front of their huts accost us and gesticulate aggressively; a group of young women waiting to fill their buckets with water are shy but add their opinions once the most assured has spoken. Water and blood are symbolically related, and when water is drunk they believe it goes into the lungs (hence people with not enough blood, with anaemia, are breathless) and from there round the body in the veins (everyone knows doctors shortcut this by pouring water into the veins direct). Measles, in turn, is within the essence of all people, and must "come out" at some time, inevitably. Vaccines are accepted with equanimity and wry suspension of disbelief in their action. Most dangerous is when the measles goes "back in"—I would explain it as severe dehydration that stops a child's tears, vomit, and diarrhoea—but we agree anyway that death may be imminent.

The ward round continues, from the successes—the child with nephrotic syndrome receiving steroids, whose smile widens daily as his swelling subsides, and the bored happy ones with broken legs hanging from pulleys— to the failures—a paralysed speechless girl brought in after fitting with meningitis for hours, whose family can no longer manage, her living skeleton malnourished and fading away despite all our efforts.

By the end of the ward round the first five or so of the day's 10 or 20 admissions are gathered. Some, at their last gasp for water or air, are given water or blood respectively. The Kenyan medical students amaze me yet again with their skill at slipping needles into the most fragile of dried out baby scalp veins; I amaze myself with a perfect lumbar puncture on a screaming urchin, and take the happily crystal-clear drops off to the laboratory. There I check the results from the day's malaria slides and write the prescriptions accordingly. After a lunch break, I wander into one of the town's cafes, the loose ends on the ward are tied up, and it is time for projects. Rob's is with the high tech transcranial Doppler ultrasound measuring blood flow in the middle cerebral artery—will this tell us important things about disease processes in very sick children? The whoosh-whoosh-whoosh pulses out at us as we walk past the little research ward.

My project is to count every drop of fluid going into and out of a child with cerebral malaria over 24 hours. Endlessly there are extra sources of error, not noticed by me as I try to add up volumes and nappy weights in the middle of the night. This year, for better and worse, the rains haven't come properly, so there is little severe malaria, and instead today I can amble back to the guesthouse, luxurious by local standards, for a swim in the balmy buoyant water. There I can dream of my next trip up the coast to the ancient Islamic island city of Lamu, an African Venice of narrow streets, donkeys, cool wind, relaxed gossip, and self indulgence by the waterside.

TA

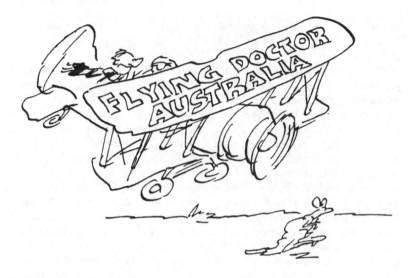

Assessments and exams

Schools adopt different systems of assessing students' clinical progress. Most combine end of attachment assessments with a final MB exam at the end of the course, which were traditionally taken in one grand slam but are increasingly now divided up into different parts over a year or longer. The final MB consists of different sections in pathology, medicine, surgery, clinical pharmacology and therapeutics, and obstetrics and gynaecology. The "minor" specialty attachments are included in the major subjects. The amount of emphasis placed on each varies, and within each the emphasis is on the ability to reason and use knowledge rather than to function as a mixture between a sponge and a parrot. Some schools prefer almost total continuous assessment with each exam contributing to the final MB. Others continue to put major emphasis on finals with the regular assessments being used to monitor progress and certify satisfactory attendance and completion of an attachment.

An increasing number of schools split finals into two, with the written papers taken a year earlier than clinicals, to encourage concentration on clinical skills and decision making before becoming a house officer.

The final MB comprises multiple choice questions, extended answers to structured questions, or essays, and practicals. In medicine (which includes paediatrics and psychiatry), surgery, and obstetrics and gynaecology considerable emphasis is placed on the clinical bedside examination, which tests skills in talking to patients, eliciting the relevant clinical signs, and making a diagnosis. Oral examinations are also held in most subjects. Clinical skills are increasingly being tested in a more systematic way through Objective Structured Clinical Exams (OSCEs). A few minutes are spent by all candidates at a series of "stations" at which they have to perform a particular task, or address a problem.

However the exams are structured, there is no avoiding the fact that they require considerable amounts of work over a prolonged period. They are as much a test of emotional stability and physical endurance as they are of knowledge and skills. Most students do pass at their first attempt; up to 10% have to resit all or part of their finals six months later. Very few fail more than once.

REMEMBER

- The later years are more like being an apprentice than a conventional student.

- The course is largely concerned with core clinical skills, strategies of investigation and treatment, and professional attitudes.

- Much of the learning is from patients, including acute emergencies, and at times it is necessary for students to live in the hospital overnight or occasionally for longer periods.

- Students may travel to nearby hospitals, community health centres and GP surgeries for a broader exposure to medical practice.

- The main clinical components are the principles and practice of general medicine and surgery and their related sub-specialties: obstetrics and gynaecology, child health, psychiatry, clinical pharmacology and therapeutics, and the underlying pathology sciences. Communication skills and ethics continue as important themes.

- Choice and opportunities for study in depth are provided through special study modules which may be expanded to lead to an intercalated science degree.

- The elective period, which most students spend abroad, is a great opportunity to travel and learn how medicine is practised in other countries and cultures.

- Assessment in the later years is by a mixture of in-course and end-of-course assessments and final examinations, testing clinical skills, attitudes and ability to use the knowledge gained. The pattern of assessment used varies substantially between schools.

- Up to 10% of students may fail one or more parts of their finals on one occasion but most are successful at a second attempt.

9. Doubts

Doubts are a very normal part of most people's lives. No university course, and no professional training, is more likely to raise doubts than medicine: academic doubts, vocational doubts, and personal doubts.

As Richard Smith, editor of the *BMJ*, once wrote:

Once they arrive, medical students are put through a gruelling course and exposed younger than most of their non-medical friends to death, pain, sickness, and what the great doctor William Osler called the perplexity of the soul. And all this within an environment where "real doctors" get on with the job and only the weak weep or feel distressed. After qualification, doctors work absurdly hard, are encouraged to tackle horrible problems with inadequate support, and then face a lifetime of pretending that they have more powers than they actually do. And all this within an environment where narcotics and the means to kill yourself are readily available. No wonder some doctors develop serious problems.

Few intending medical students never have reservations whether medicine is right for them and they for medicine. All too often these doubts have concentrated too much on the process of getting into medical school and too little on what being a doctor is all about, the consequence of which being to add to the cynicism and disillusionment which is rife among junior doctors. After working for several years on the BBC TV series *Doctors To Be*, the producer Susan Spindler recognised this problem and offered some good advice:

It's hard to take a career decision at the age of 17; at that age many people haven't quite decided who they are and many of us change almost beyond recognition between the ages of 17 and 25. If you are in any doubt about your suitability for the medical life, postpone the decision: do another degree first and wait until you are certain before entering medicine. Even if you've been set on becoming a doctor since you were a young child, do your homework first: spend time with as many doctors as you can—in hospitals and surgeries, doing different kinds of jobs. Get a clear idea of the range of possibilities that medicine can offer.

Once at medical school not many students survive five years without wondering if they are on the right track. Doctors in the early years after qualification are almost universally nagged with doubts about finding jobs, obtaining higher qualifications, and whether their aspirations are realistic in terms of skills and opportunities.

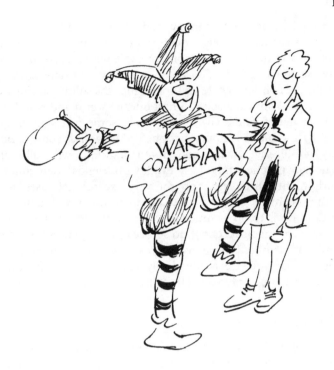

Alongside these academic and vocational doubts the world of doctors in training also creaks and groans with all the normal difficulties of men and women finding their feet in an adult world. If newly away from home they must find accommodation and adjust to the responsibilities that brings. Mature students must acclimatise to a world that is often very different, more hierarchical, and more juvenile than that in which their feet have been so firmly planted for some years. Coping with the financial difficulties, experienced by most students but particularly self funding mature students, can take its toll. Medical students are not immune to all the usual identity crises that strike most other students at some stage nor the relationship dramas. In some ways the pressure to conform that pervades medicine in general, and in medical schools in particular, does nothing to make such problems easier; the pressure on time, especially at exam times and in the early years after qualification, can test even the strongest of personal involvements.

Academic doubts

Academic doubts at medical school are common in the early years. As the first set of exams or assessments approaches most students feel nervous about the amount of work they should be undertaking. The subject matter and the style of learning and of exams may be very different from previous experience. The greater emphasis on self directed learning with less of the spoon feeding by teachers that many students are used to from school can be bewildering at first. It is also much more difficult initially to gauge the amount of work to do from seeing other people working. As at school there will always seem to be individuals who sail through exams with apparent ease on minimal revision, while you spend months solidly slaving away just to scrape a pass. You will also soon find out the weird and wonderful ways some of your new friends have of studying. Some will stay up all night, others will have done four hours work before breakfast, some seem to stay up all day and all night, while one of your flatmates will still seem to be going to hockey practice, then for a drink with friends, then coming home for an early night. Of course, only the very exceptional cases do as little work as they seem to, and the best way to dispel any doubts as to how much work to do is to do as much as you can; the vast majority of people who fail exams at medical school do so because they do too little too late. You should remember you have already proved with your entrance requirements that you are academically capable of getting through the course, provided you apply yourself realistically to the task ahead.

Vocational doubts

Doubts of a very different nature often surface when you are faced with dealing with patients. Often this is because of the perception of the student that their need to learn from the patient without really contributing directly to their management makes them feel they are intruding and that the patient is resentful of their involvement. This is rarely the case, and a student with more time to spend talking than busy junior doctors can make a considerable contribution to the care of patients, most of whom also fully recognise that we all have to learn somewhere and on someone. One patient described her experience like this.

My student

There must come a time when books and lectures need to be supplemented with real experience on real patients. Most people are happy to oblige; after all they are altruistic enough to give blood and carry organ donor cards, and it's more agreeable to give students access to your live body than to donate it for "spare parts".

I was first examined by students during one of my pregnancies. I had to rest in hospital for several weeks and was captive for any passing student to listen to my heart murmur and my baby's heart: two for the price of one.

Recently I was in hospital again. The relationship between student and patient can be mutually beneficial. The student can be a comforting presence, having more time to spend with the patient than the busy registrar on his or her brisk ward round, and the student's attention is a welcome break in the crushing boredom of life in a hospital ward. Do not underestimate the importance of a student's interest in a patient. Other patients watch enviously as the curtains are swished closed round your bed, ears strain to hear what is going on inside.

My student last time was a girl and quite young. She was extremely polite, with a warm friendly approach which helped me to relax. My permission was sought and I agreed to let her examine me, literally from head to toe. I touched my nose; my eyes followed her pen as she moved it across my visual field; I wriggled my toes for her, I must confess to a feeling of slight amusement as she consulted her highlighted textbook as we completed each test. She even admitted that it was the first time she had done this. I was quite touched.

My student had to take my medical history and present it to the rest of the team. She seemed to be very thorough, much more thorough than an earlier student in her final year. She was relaxed and spoke confidently about my case and having done her homework answered all the questions that were fired at her. I felt she did well and that she already has a good bedside manner.

Occasionally it is possible to recognise a former student after they have qualified. I was visiting a patient in hospital when this happened. The doctor came to see the patient, and as she turned to go she actually remembered me; I was so pleased. I could not help noticing that gone was her slightly hesitant student manner, apologising for having cold hands; in its place was a brisk confident doctor doing a great job in a busy hospital. How proud I felt to have played a small part.

BS

Learning from patients, especially in the early years, can occasionally be disturbing and unsettling. Coming to terms with blood, disfigurement, suffering, disability, mental illness, incurable disease, and death is difficult for all students, but most will overcome it without becoming hard and completely detached. A few others find it hard to relate to patients, which is then compounded by them failing to develop the essential skills in talking to and examining patients. Usually the best remedy in these cases is to engineer a greater degree of involvement and responsibility, but with more and better communication skills teaching in schools now such students can find a good deal of help available. Occasionally this gulf seems unbridgeable, and the student may have to decide whether to change course or to press on to qualification in the knowledge that many careers in medicine have limited contact with patients.

Personal doubts

The number of young doctors leaving medicine is nothing like as high as has been reported. Fewer than 5% change career in the first five years after qualification. Any loss at this stage represents a substantial waste of public money; but, more than that, any waste of bright, talented, motivated, dedicated individuals with ideals and aspirations which led them to become

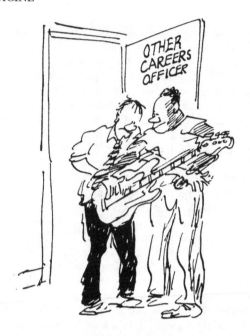

doctors in the first place and who, for whatever reasons, decide to give up is a tragedy. The factors which lead to disillusionment in young doctors are numerous (even if they do not leave medicine), and many of the issues, particularly over long hours, have now been dealt with, with some success. Some of the problem, however, lies with the junior doctors themselves. Too many doctors admit they did not know what they were letting themselves in for. Nor perhaps did they realise the limitations of medicine to meet the high expectations of the public—or of themselves. The earlier the problem is examined the better: perhaps the combination of an improvement in working conditions and a generation of enlightened, well informed new doctors with an understanding of what lies ahead will lead to better morale and less waste.

Given the breadth of talent of most successful applicants to medical school it should come as little surprise that a major concern for many doctors is that they have "sold their soul to medicine" and are now incapable of doing anything else. In reality, many simply feel trapped in a job they begin to resent. They feel they have lost, or had knocked out of them, all the dreams and potential they had when they arrived at medical school. An old Chinese aphorism states, "You grow old not by having birthdays, but by deserting ideals", and being a tired, harassed, stressed junior doctor makes you feel prematurely old. Perhaps there is much that can be done within the structure of medicine to prevent "burn out" but doctors sometimes need reminding that "the grass is always greener ...".

There is no escaping the fact that medicine is not just a job but a way of life. It is important to realise that far from being less likely than others to have serious problems, doctors are in some ways more likely to. They need to be prepared to discuss their problems and to seek appropriate help. Susan Spindler, producer of the *Doctors To Be* series had this to say about doubts and some ways of dealing with them:

> The early years as a qualified doctor can be so tough that they test the strongest of vocations. A supportive network of family and friends—people on whom you can offload anxieties and with whom you can share traumatic experiences—can make the difference between staying and quitting. You need all the student qualities listed above [see pp. 23–25] plus initiative and the ability to take decisions. A robust value system that isn't driven by the pursuit of riches—you'll probably see school and university peers working far shorter hours for far more money during your late 20s and early 30s. A need to compromise on the wish to achieve all you can in your career *and* forge a relationship/marriage and raise a family—a particular source of difficulty for women in hospital medicine. A supportive partner or spouse certainly makes life much easier. And, if you have managed to keep a circle of non-medical friends, you'll reap the rewards now: many doctors find themselves trapped in a world of medical politics and socialising—it's much easier to maintain a balanced view of life if some of the people you spend time with are not doctors.

Vocational doubts and academic failures occasionally occur during the course because of psychiatric illness, which is sometimes the outcome of relentless parental pressure to follow a career which a student either did not want or for which he or she was unsuited. Depression is the usual response. Expert advice is needed. Psychiatric illness may be self limiting but it may be persistent or recurrent and incompatible with the standards of service and judgment which patients have a right to expect.

The importance of seeking help and advice before problems become overwhelming cannot be too strongly emphasised. Most difficulties tend to grow if incubated. In the first place there is no substitute for sharing problems with good friends, and that is one reason why a successful school needs to be a happy, considerate community and not just an academic factory. But the advice of friends may need to be supplemented by tutors, other teachers, doctors in the students' health service, pastors, priests, or parents. Although it is true that a problem shared is a problem halved, a problem anticipated can be a problem avoided. No problems are unique and none insuperable. Very occasionally the right move is to change course, in which case the sooner the better. To change direction for good reason is the beginning of a new opportunity, not a disaster.

One thing is reasonably certain: decisions either to learn medicine or to abandon the task should not be taken too quickly. As Lilian Hellman wrote in *The Little Foxes*: "Sometimes it's better to let the sun rise again."

REMEMBER

- Doubts are a normal part of everyone's life.

- Most doubts are about personal ability and career aspirations.

- Mature students, more than most, have moments when they question whether they are doing the right thing.

- Anyone who has achieved the entry requirements to medical school need have no doubts about academic ability. Academic failure normally only results from working too little, too late, and in a disorganised way.

- The few who will have doubts about relating to patients can be helped through communication skills training.

- Unrealistic expectations can lead to doubts but can be avoided, and prevention lies in an honest appraisal of oneself and careful researching before opting for the career.

- Occasionally the decision to enter medicine turns out to be a mistake. Changing course or career is a brave move which can lead to a new and more fulfilling life.

- The best remedy for doubts is to share them with someone; you will find you are not alone.

10. The house officer

Almost all medical students would agree that the final exams for the qualification of Bachelor of Medicine and Bachelor of Surgery, whatever the precise form they take, are the most terrifying and daunting experience of their lives. That is until a few weeks later when they walk onto the wards for the first time as a "proper doctor". After six years of preparing for this day you are thrust headlong into the real world. To become a really proper doctor, that is to be a fully registered medical practitioner, the General Medical Council (GMC) requires a new doctor to complete a year of satisfactory service in recognised, appropriately supervised preregistration house officer posts.

The real world

In a white coat, never again to be so clean and tidy, with pockets bulging with books, pens, notepads, and all manner of equipment you have little idea how to use, you walk proudly on to your ward to be met by an enigmatic look from the formidable Sister that expresses exasperation and pity all rolled into one. A couple of hours later the sparkle of youthful enthusiasm has been transformed into a downcast look of dread mixed with horror. You have been introduced, albeit fleetingly, to your team, and one of them actually said hello, or at least that was what you had assumed the registrar meant when he growled at you.

Now for the patients. There are quite a few at the moment because the team was on call at the weekend and it has become really busy since they closed down the old infirmary up the road. You frantically try to write down everything your predecessor is telling you, even though you have not a clue what she means by half of it, and you haven't time to ask any questions because she is in a rush to get to her new job in the Shetland Islands, which she was due to start three hours ago. Then your bleep goes off: a patient to see in the accident and emergency department; he has already waited half an hour and he's shouting about the "Patient's Charter". Then you have to go for your computer induction course but can't find where it is. You also need to go to the toilet but you can't find that either. And your consultant's secretary has just rung you to tell you to take some notes to your boss in the outpatient clinic. On the way you find a scruffy looking elderly gentleman slumped in the corner of the lift. Is he drunk or just asleep? You are fairly sure he is actually breathing, but just in case you get out at the next floor and use the stairs. Your bleep goes again: Mrs Smith needs some paracetamol, but you don't know the dose; Mr Jones needs a new drip siting, and you always missed the vein as a student, at least he didn't need a catheter, you have never even attempted one of those, never mind a successful one. And Mr Patel's son has arrived and wants to talk to a doctor. And there is still that man in A&E, and the consultant also wants an *x* ray fetched from the boot of his Volvo.

It is now four o'clock in the afternoon, no lunch yet and come to think of it you still haven't found the toilet. Your registrar is now waiting on the ward to go round all the patients to check you have finished all the jobs from this morning. Never mind, you are on call tonight, so only another 26 hours at work and then you can go home.

Suddenly after six years in the sanctuary of the medical school, this is the real world, the world of what is officially called a house officer, but is more generally called a houseman—regardless of sex—or even, more or less affectionately, "housepixies", "housedogs", or "houseplants".

SS

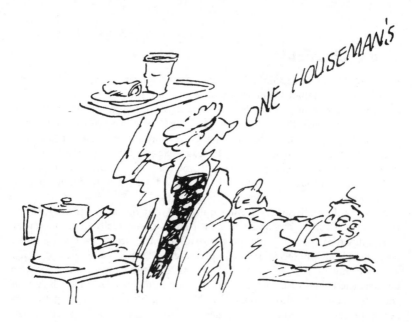

Preregistration year

House jobs are almost always undertaken immediately after qualifying, and it is not a good idea to take time off at this stage, such as for travelling or further study; better to get the year over and done with while all you have learned is fresh in your mind.

The year is usually split into two six month posts: one in a medical specialty, which includes the care of medical emergencies of all sorts and often includes some time working in a care of the elderly unit, and one in a surgical specialty, which involves the care of acutely ill patients with surgical emergencies, with special experience, for example, in orthopaedics, urology, or vascular surgery. Increasingly, rotations are being introduced which involve four months in general practice along with four months each in medicine and surgery in hospital. Some new schemes include paediatrics or gynaecology in place of general practice.

The houseman is the bottom rung of the medical ladder; it is no less important for that. The houseman is normally based on the wards, providing the regular, front line contact between the patients and the team of doctors looking after them. Much of the time is spent talking to new patients about the details of their illness (taking a history) and examining them, ordering the initial investigations and collecting the results, carrying out the management plan worked out with the more senior members of the team, and coping with day to day problems such as pain control, fluid balance, and organising discharge and follow up arrangements.

The houseman's role requires good communication skills. Whether it is listening to the patient's story of their illness and drawing out all the information needed to make an accurate diagnosis; explaining the patient's condition, treatment or progress; offering reassurance; or breaking bad news when appropriate. While this is for many new doctors the hardest part of their job, and often the one for which medical school has in the past least prepared them, the intimacy of the doctor–patient relationship can be thoroughly rewarding, if occasionally harrowing, like the patient dying of renal cancer who told her houseman that his care and kindness was making dying less frightening and lonely than she had expected.

In addition to the daytime work, a houseman is on call, usually on a rota of one in six nights and weekends, living in the hospital to provide emergency care for the patients on the wards and any new patients who need to be admitted to hospital. In most cases, when as a houseman you have worked a night, sometimes all night, you are expected to be at work as normal the next day. You should be able to go off after the "post-take" ward round, reviewing all the new patients with the consultant and registrar, and after having tied up the loose ends of treatment, investigations, and discharge, but this can take most of the day. On some firms the houseman goes off at 10 am the next morning but then does not see what happens to the patients admitted during the night and so misses the chance to learn from the experience. This is very different from working night shifts like nurses, for example, and is something almost all housemen find difficult to cope with, especially in busy jobs. The dreadful feeling at 4 am of finally climbing into your bed and reaching across to put out the light and hearing the bleep go off again, summoning you back to the ward you had just left, is something you will never forget. It is quite amazing how your bleep seems to know exactly the wrong times to go off, such as just as you sit

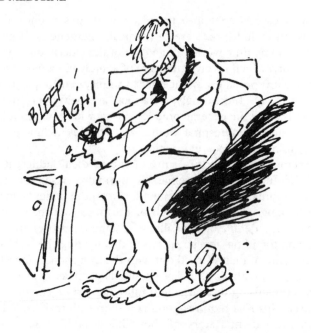

down with the sandwich you have just managed to grab between seeing patients, or just as you have stepped into the shower, or every time you try to go to the toilet.

Every houseman has stories of how annoying some of these calls are, such as the call from a nurse at 2 am to ask if she should wake up Mr Smith to give him his sleeping pill, or the call at 5 am by the staff nurse just showing a student how the bleep system worked. My "favourite" was the patient I was called to see in the middle of the night because he was cold and shivering. Concerned he may have developed a dangerous fever I raced from my room across the snowy car park, my mind racing for possible causes, only to find on my arrival a poor old soul lying in a bed with no blankets and next to a window which was wide open to the freezing December weather. "Six years at medical school just to close a bloody window" was the comment I was heard muttering under my breath as I stomped off back to bed.

Rotas or shifts

Some hospitals have introduced partial shift systems for their junior staff, where a houseman may work three weeks of days followed by a week of nights or may find they work split weekend shifts, so that the periods of continuous on call are reduced. Often the intensity of work is much greater and the disruption of shift work, both on continuity of patient care and doctors' personal lives, arguably outweighs many of the benefits of more protected sleep time. These shifts vary greatly between hospitals and

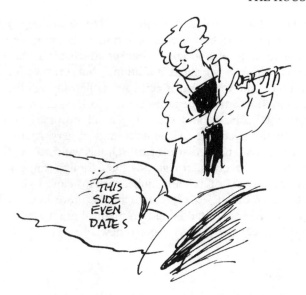

departments and consequently vary in their popularity among staff and patients. On call arrangements are changing all the time, and it is worth keeping in touch with developments in this area as before too long it may have an important impact on your life. For example, many hospitals have arrangements that all housemen go to bed at midnight when they are on call and the senior house officers cover any emergencies at night. In other hospitals, physicians' assistants have been employed who can perform many of the routine tasks that housemen are usually expected to do, such as filling in basic forms, taking blood samples, and re-siting intravenous drips.

In theory the preregistration posts complete basic medical education and training, with the houseman effectively on loan from the university to the NHS. The long hours and heavy workload, often including tasks more appropriate to non-medical staff, however, has in the past meant that this training aspect of the job has been neglected. Much has recently been done to attempt to reduce junior doctors' hours and to limit repetitive tasks of little educational value, with a formal structure for meeting and monitoring the educational and training needs of housemen. Much more can still be done, but all housemen should now expect to receive protected time for formal teaching and a named tutor throughout their attachments.

With the initiatives from the government to reduce junior doctors' hours, housemen should not be on duty for more than an average of 72 hours a week (including time on call), with not more than 56 hours actually worked and continuous duty—for example, over a weekend on call not exceeding 32 hours. In practice, some doctors are still working on rotas which are non-compliant with the latest New Deal for junior doctors. Regional Pre-Registration House Officer Sub-Deans and New Deal Task Forces are monitoring these conditions much more closely than ever before, largely through doctors completing compulsory work diaries. Hospitals can face stiff financial penalties if their doctors are found to be working inappropriate duties or if conditions such as accommodation or catering are inadequate.

As with the training of housemen there is much more that can and is being done to improve working conditions, but prospective housemen should keep up to date with what is going on, either through the press or by talking to current housemen when they are on work experience attachments.

Most teaching hospitals and district general hospitals employ house officers in the major specialties of medicine and surgery. Many of these are linked in schemes with particular medical schools which try to find jobs for as many of their new graduates as possible, though some new doctors prefer to find their own "off scheme" jobs, perhaps close to home or where they hope to settle down. At present there are more house officer posts available than there are United Kingdom medical graduates, so every new graduate is effectively guaranteed a job somewhere.

Where to go

The experience gained in different types of hospitals varies greatly—for example, between a small rural district hospital, which may offer a better exposure to common, "bread and butter" medical conditions, and a large inner city teaching hospital, which may have a much narrower range of patients but with a chance of exposure to research and the most modern technology. Prospective housemen look for jobs most suited to their interests and career intentions, with most trying to achieve some variety and balance. For example, an aspiring young surgeon may decide to do his or her surgical house job in a high profile academic unit then a medical job in a district general hospital, while a would-be general practitioner may choose to do both jobs in a district general hospital in an area he or she wants to practise in eventually. Often other factors are taken into account: a keen surfer or sailor may well choose a job near the coast while an inner city job may be more preferable for the keen theatre goer or night clubber! Some people have special ties, for example, a spouse with or without children who cannot readily move just for six months or even a season ticket for the local football club.

Like most jobs in medicine, the preregistration house officer year (PRHO) is extremely demanding, perhaps not intellectually, but certainly physically and emotionally. The down sides are well known—long hours, little sleep, poor conditions, unfamiliarity with the job, and little recognition. Although the situation is improving, it is still not uncommon for even the strongest character to be put sorely to the test during this time, with the butchest rugby forward being reduced to tears, not to mention the ladies' hockey goalkeeper. At times like this the friendships and camaraderie that typify medical students are worth their weight in gold.

It is not all doom and gloom though. The houseman is uniquely placed to be able to develop good doctor–patient relationships, to be involved in close teamwork, putting the last six years of theory into practice, and, not least, to have the feeling of actually being needed and being useful: something you hardly ever feel as a medical student. The pay cheque at the end of the month is, of course, rather welcome too but will not bowl you over.

It is interesting to note that while in the midst of their year most housemen see their posts as a means to an end, something to be endured which will soon be over; once they are over, however, and the doctor has moved on to bigger and better things, a surprising number of them look back on being a houseman as the happiest days, and nights, of their lives.

REMEMBER

- After passing finals and graduating in medicine all doctors are required to spend a year of supervised experience as a house officer.

- Your medical degree qualifies you for provisional registration with the General Medical Council. Successful completion of your house officer posts entitles you to full registration.

- The year must contain both medicine and surgery, including care of acute emergencies. Some posts containing general practice or other specialties are increasingly available.

- House officers are normally not permitted to be on duty for an average of more than 72 hours per week of which 56 hours is actual work, allowing for rest periods while on call in the hospital; you should not undertake more than 32 hours of continuous duty (56 at weekends) during which you are entitled to at least eight hours' rest. In practice, an appreciable number of junior doctors are still having to work longer or more intensively, and this is still a major cause of contention in the NHS.

- House officers are the first line in the medical team, and are responsible for the day-to-day care of patients (under supervision), and the organisation of investigations and treatment. Communication with patients and their relatives is a crucial part of the role.

- The type of job and its location depends partly on personal preferences and career intentions.

- Being a house officer is one of the hardest years of your life. It is disruptive of your personal life, physically and emotionally demanding, and leaves almost everyone close to tears at least once in the year. It can also show teamwork at its best, be good training, great fun, and immensely fulfilling.

11. Choosing a specialty

A candidate was asked at his medical school interview where he saw himself in, say, 20 years hence. "I want to be a brain surgeon," was the 17 year old's confident reply. Few medical students, and indeed newly qualified doctors, could be quite so sure of their career intentions. Choosing a specialty provides many young medics with the seemingly endless dilemmas of balancing employment opportunities, specialty preferences, personal and family circumstances, and choosing where, when and with whom to settle down.

It is important to remember you are not alone in being undecided, you are allowed to change your mind, you are allowed a life outside your career, and eventually most doctors find their niche and have a happy, fulfilled life and career.

Some specialties are much more difficult than others to reconcile with family commitments or other interests, especially in the early postgraduate years. Some can say with Dawn Adamson, recently qualified at the time, "I don't see being a doctor as a job—I see it as a way of life." But others can also be good doctors while keeping medicine in its place. Keeping medicine in its place can be difficult and Julian Eyers, also a recent graduate, was right to point out that public (and professional) expectations of doctors may fail to recognise that doctors are human too: he referred to "… a public misconception that doctors are some sort of breed apart of medical soldiers, ready to be drafted into any situation. Doctors are actually human beings. They have loved ones, emotions, and outside lives. The conditions are frequently so inhuman that they take an unacceptable toll on their private and professional lives!"

Not only a parent or the carer of elderly relatives, but also the dedicated sportsman, musician, or enthusiast for a full life may wonder whether an otherwise attractive specialty would unacceptably monopolise their lives and stifle their interests. Given the structure of society and the traditionally predominant responsibility of the mother for the family, many of the issues particularly concern women in medicine, but many male doctors have family responsibilities too and other time consuming interests.

Long hours, resident on call duties, and shift arrangements designed to reduce hours but creating their own problems in turn, both for structured life and for systematic postgraduate education, are at the centre of the conflict. Doctors in accident and emergency departments usually work a

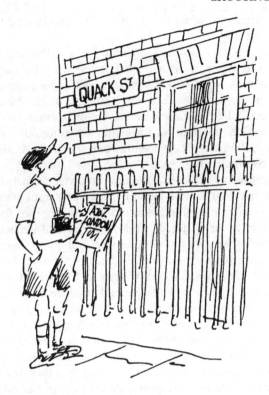

round the clock shift system, which involves a predictable and regular commitment. Some other departments are beginning to work a partial shift system, with several weeks on days interspersed with a week on night duty. Other departments are forming larger teams to reduce the night and weekend on call duties, within an otherwise traditional rota system. The maximum permitted average contracted hours of duty for doctors in training is now 56 hours a week, equivalent to being on call about one in six if you are also responsible for covering colleagues when on holiday, study leave, or during brief illness.

Becoming a thoroughly fulfilled doctor is compatible with domestic commitments provided both partners are prepared to share fully the task of house and home. The trouble is that more than half of married doctors are themselves married to doctors, with all the difficulty that that entails, including coordinating on call duties, finding geographically convenient higher specialist training programmes, and eventually obtaining mutually compatible career posts. There may simply not be two appropriate posts in suitable locations within a reasonable time. If both partners are in the same specialty the possibility of job sharing might arise. General practice is a better bet than a hospital-based specialty, not least because home and practice are often close together. One couple, for example, took over a single handed country practice and successfully shared both the practice and the home duties. Their patients benefited from continuity of care from a close knit partnership, while the doctors' own children had the attention of both their parents.

There are several reasons why women are less well represented in some specialties than in others. For one thing, some specialties appeal more to men than women. Another is that some specialties are more demanding in their unsocial hours and therefore more difficult to combine with regular domestic responsibilities which bear harder on women. Women tend to choose non-surgical specialties, with the exception of ophthalmology. Paediatrics and public health are the only two specialties initially chosen by women more commonly than men.

Both men and women doctors take time to arrive at their final choice of specialty and most do not think very much about it until after they qualify. Towards the end of the preregistration period choices for paediatrics, general medicine, general surgery, and obstetrics and gynaecology exceed opportunity. Preferences for pathology and radiology are about matched to opportunity, and psychiatry, general practice, and public health are undersubscribed. However, fashions change all the time in medical careers, and there is a move back towards general practice in some parts of the country, but job opportunities still exceed those wishing to take them up. Over the subsequent few years 25–33% of doctors change their choices, some more than once. About 40% of the changes of preference (and about 60% in women with children) are because of family commitments. Specialties such as general practice now come into their own, being more readily compatible with other responsibilities, both in flexibility of working practice and in the earlier attainment of a settled home and secure income. Hospital specialties which allow other commitments either through well organised duty rotas or light on call responsibility or by providing good opportunities for part time work include anaesthetics, accident and emergency, psychiatry, pathology, radiology, oncology, medicine for the elderly, rehabilitation medicine, and medical specialties such as dermatology, genitourinary medicine, and palliative care. Public health also offers regular and reasonable hours. Overall, a recent survey showed that half of women and a quarter of men considered marriage to have been a constraint on their career in medicine. Eventually, preconceived ambitions have to be balanced against the practicalities of personal commitments and professional training. In this, medicine is by no means unique.

A determined effort is being made to introduce good opportunities for "flexible training", but more still needs to be done to reduce the conflict between family responsibilities and a career in medicine and to diminish the relatively greater disadvantage of women. As Yvonne Noble, a sociologist, has written:

> Adjustments in the profession must be inevitable: when the adjustments are made it is essential that they do not continue to disadvantage those (men as well as women) who recognise their need for and responsibility to personal partners and children.

Practical measures being introduced include widespread provision of crèches in the NHS and a means through tax allowances, of offsetting the costs of assistance with child care. Better career advice is needed, both at medical school and in the early postgraduate years, but it may be of rather limited value until the circumstances of personal life unfold. Most doctors eventually find their way through the maze but they and their families deserve more readily available signposts and smoother paths to a permanent post.

When should you decide

Some fortunate people decide on their careers as students (fortunate, that is, if they have made a realistic decision), more decide as house officers, and most decide in the next year or two while undertaking general professional training in senior house officer posts. Many senior house officer posts are not part of a specialist training programme but offer general training and experience. They are vital feet-finding posts. Most students qualify with little idea of the wide range of career opportunities open to them, an ignorance which reflects badly both on medical schools for not opening their students' eyes and on students themselves for often lacking curiosity about their own future. The hurdles of finals and house jobs completely dominate their thinking.

Careers fairs are held annually in many parts of the country to display the attractions of different specialties and to offer advice from doctors in all major specialties on a personal and informal level. Advice is available in medical schools from postgraduate sub-deans and in each district general hospital from the clinical tutor or director of postgraduate medical education and training. Each region of the NHS also has a regional postgraduate dean who is responsible for overall coordination of postgraduate training and career advice, supported by individual assistant deans with special responsibility for each phase and area of postgraduate medical education and training. Each Royal College also appoints regional advisers and hospital Royal College tutors to whom trainees can turn.

Career decisions depend on many factors, but a clear idea of the wide opportunities available is the first necessity. Most teachers of clinical medicine are hospital physicians or surgeons who wittingly, or unwittingly, give the impression that these are the only two worthy careers. House officer posts are also dominated by these specialties. Consequently, for years too many doctors have wanted to specialise in hospital specialties such as general medicine and general surgery and too few in, for example, pathology, psychiatry, geriatrics, and mental handicap. Most doctors, whether deciding to work in or out of hospital, prefer to live in green pastures not in inner cities. Until 15 years ago general practice was not a common first choice. It then became very popular but currently recruitment is not keeping pace with demand. Many see general practice as more compatible than hospital specialties with a life of their own. At the end of the day, not every doctor ends up in their specialty of first choice because, in the words of George Bernard Shaw: "Up to a certain point doctors, like carpenters and masons, must earn their living by doing work that the public wants from them." Or, put another way by the chief medical officer of the Department of Health: "The aim of undergraduate medical education is to produce doctors who are able to meet the present and future need of the health services."

Medicine is, however, a mine of opportunity. A range of different specialties beckons all sorts of personalities and interests. Most of these specialties are "clinical", they primarily serve individuals; they do much for a few and are in reserve for many. Other specialties, by contrast, are population rather than person based; they do much for many and seek health for all. Doctors in all specialties, whether focused primarily on individuals or populations, have some way still to go in persuading the public to take responsibility for preserving their own health.

Medicine is many things but nothing if not a service, in Britain a national health service. The original vision which created it is very much alive, despite relentless financial, organisational, and ethical pressures associated with an aging population and advancing medical technology. Medicine and the NHS have also never before been so much in the spotlight of the national media, adding even more pressures to staff. A combination of good clinical common sense, public restraint, and appropriate prioritisation of national resources can still ensure that, as originally announced in 1944:

> ... every man, woman and child can rely on getting all the advice, treatment and care which they need in matters of personal health: that what they will get will be the best medicine and other facilities available: that their getting them should not depend on whether they can pay for them or on any factor irrelevant to the real need—the real need to bring the country's full resources to bear upon reducing ill health and promoting good health for all its citizens. ...

at least as far as a health service alone can achieve good health for all.

Perfect fits are for machines; more roughly crafted men and women and evolving specialties are seldom made precisely for each other. But if the interest and the will are there, the individual and the specialty can develop together like partners in a successful marriage. Doctor and specialty is not the only fit which matters. Spare a thought for the doctor–patient relationship on the way, bearing in mind Dr Brotschi's snapshots of "the kind of doctors we shouldn't be" in a letter to the *New England Journal of Medicine*:

> First, the ambitious climber take,
> Who will the department chairman make;
> Who toils to win Professors' praise
> And quotes the Journal, phrase by phrase,
> But never reads the patients' gaze.

Next: the expert proud we find,
The latest saviour to mankind.
Cured patients speak to his renown,
But he leaves sick ones with a frown,
Because they let his image down.

Third, the jovial friend of all,
Who never heard perfection's call.
His ken of medicine paper thin,
But patients' trust he'll always win:
They love him while he does them in.

And fourth, the well adjusted fellow,
Who seeks that all in life be mellow;
Who loves good music, wine and skis,
Resents his work but likes the fees,
And does not hear his patients' pleas.

To start the series, here are four,
But surely there are many more,
Just let us seek and see what's true
In what we are and what we do,
Lest we forget, we're human too.

Every doctor becomes a specialist, even in something as general sounding as general practice, perhaps better called "family medicine", which is as much a special art as any other part of medical practice. Becoming a specialist may not seem that difficult, judged from the bogus doctors who have remained undetected not just for a casual day or two, which is not all that uncommon, but for years. A 64 year old man with a stolen medical degree was sentenced at Leeds Crown Court after working for 30 years as a general practitioner. Amazingly, neither his patients (who demonstrated outside the court room in his support), nor his colleagues rumbled him. A pharmacist in the chemist next door to the surgery raised the alarm, not perhaps before time. "If one 5 ml spoonful of hair shampoo is to be taken three times a day", the pharmacist told the court, "You tend to think there is something wrong. Time and again there were inhalers to be injected, tablets to be rubbed in—all very unusual". Very unusual!

General practice is not the only home of bogus doctors. Amaedeo Goria of Canelli near Turin, practised for 13 years as a neurologist before he was "unwittingly betrayed by his adoring wife after telling her one lie too many about his professional prowess". She passed on to the local newspaper his story that he had brilliantly passed an examination in Rome, which qualified him to become head of the neurology service at the local hospital. This news sparked off an inquiry which revealed to the contrary that he was a failed medical student who had forged his diploma.

It could be said that both profession and public need their gullible heads examined, but they would be wise to take care who does it. About the same

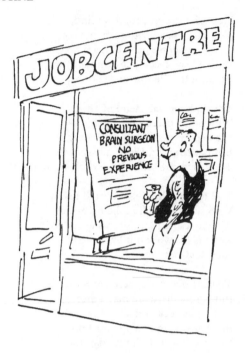

time as Goria was unmasked, another failed medical student in Italy was discovered, not because of surgical incompetence but because of "corruption in appointing senior medical personnel". He had practised for 10 years as a neurosurgeon without detection.

What makes a specialist

Specialties are a complex web of medical and surgical strands, of individual and population focus, and of hospital and community base. They interweave and overlap and can be excellently practised only by doctors who know more than their own specialty both in broad approach to difficult diagnosis and in management of the whole person. They also need to have a perspective on the sometimes conflicting interests of individual patients and the population as a whole. Specialists need to be more than two dimensional cardboard cutouts blown over by the first unfamiliar breeze. That is why it is fundamental that basic medical education and training paints a picture of the whole canvas of health, disease, and human behaviour, producing a doctor generally equipped to move into any specialty, a product once described as "the uncommitted iatroblast". That is why the preregistration house officer year is designed to develop clinical skills with both a medical and a surgical perspective and why moves are being made not only to balance the specialty base but the context by including a period in general practice within the preregistration year.

The need to be able to think and work across specialty boundaries is not new. The *Lancet* in 1827 quoted Mr Lawrence's introductory lecture to the spring course of surgery at the New Theatre in Aldersgate, London:

> Thus, whatever course we take we arrive at the same conclusion, viz that they are merely parts of one science and art; that the scientific principles are the same and the same means must be used both by the physician and the surgeon, because they have the same ends to accomplish. ... A French minister seems to have judged pretty correctly of the matter. The propriety of separating physic and surgery was strongly represented to him; "I would elevate", said the advocate of the measure "A wall of brass between them". "Pray Sir", rejoined the minister, "On which side of the wall do you propose to place the patients?".

Senior house officer posts

While the preregistration year is designed to consolidate and develop further a broad range of clinical skills of wide application, the senior house officer period was originally introduced to give a broad introduction and foundation in a particular specialty area—medicine, surgery, obstetrics and gynaecology, pathology, etc, in such a way as to enable the recent graduate to discover whether somewhere within that specialty lay the career choice for him or her. This usually involved an uncoordinated series of posts with a new application to be made every six months, often in a different part of the country as programmes of linked posts were few and far between. Some doctors undertook this period of general professional training in the armed services on a short service commission, and a few doctors made arrangements to take approved posts overseas. If the specialty first tried was not congenial, it was possible to use the training as a background for general practice or as part of training in another specialty.

Senior house officer posts are now becoming more specialised and therefore less suitable both for general training and as uncommitted career thinking time. On the other hand, most are now linked together in a designed sequence over about two years, avoiding the scramble for one job after another. In some countries, specialty streaming starts in the undergraduate course; in China, for example, students heading for careers in paediatrics or public health take a different undergraduate clinical course from other students.

While pressure to start specialisation early may be understandable in terms of shortening training and concentrating expertise, it fails to recognise the fundamental importance of a broad base as the foundation of specialist education and training. As Dr Holly Smith, an American dean of medicine, expressed it:

> ... in education as in biology, early differentiation (specialisation) leads to maturation but not necessarily to growth. This premature type of differentiation is like giving thyroxin to a tadpole. You get an instant frog but unfortunately a rather small one.

Although the broad pattern of specialty training is becoming standardised, the nature of the work and the higher qualifications required are quite different in each specialty. Some specialties, such as general medicine, general surgery, paediatrics, and obstetrics and gynaecology, are in the front line of emergency care of patients and involve substantial resident duties at nights and weekends (and are correspondingly better paid at junior level than training posts in specialties such as pathology and public health, which offer regular hours and no resident on call duties). At consultant level, the basic NHS pay is the same in all specialties and extra duty payments are not made. The opportunities for supplementing NHS income in private practice in an agreed fraction of the consultant's time are, however, much better in some specialties (mostly surgical) and in some parts of the country (mainly large cities and in particular London).

Preparation for all specialties, including public health, has now become semistructured and organised, leading to registration as a specialist after about five years of higher training, which begins two or three years after qualification as a doctor. Specialist education is largely an apprenticeship based on the everyday service responsibilities. More closely supervised training is helping to overcome the criticism of a distinguished professor that "experience, like age, receives more respect than its inevitability justifies". The shorter period of specialist training and the shorter working week for doctors in training have introduced a conflict between the length of specialist training and the acquisition of sufficient experience. An editorial in the *BMJ* observed that "between them, the New Deal [on reducing junior doctors' hours] and the Calman Report [on the length of specialist training] are reducing the time available to train a surgeon from 13 years at over 100 hours a week to eight years at 56 hours a week, a reduction of nearly two thirds" and went on to say that "under these constraints, consultants will have to extract even more teaching value from every case". Surgery may be an extreme example but the principle affects all specialties.

Membership of Royal Colleges

The Royal Colleges and specialist faculties determine standards of practice and education in the specialties. They inspect and assess both training programmes and placements. A syllabus outlines the broad areas of knowledge, skills, and attitudes required. Regular assessments by consultants nominated as clinical supervisors or tutors check the doctors' progress. Examinations for the membership or fellowship (Table 11.1) of a Royal College are taken during or, in medical specialties, before entering the specialist registrar grade. In most specialties, part I of the Royal College exams is taken early in the period of specialist training and part II serves as an exit qualification. Many doctors also take a higher university degree— MD or DM (Doctor of Medicine), awarded for a dissertation which is usually based on clinical research in the course of postgraduate training or MS or MChir (Master of Surgery), the surgical equivalent.

Table 11.1—Major professional higher qualifications

Diploma	Full title
MRCP*	Member of the Royal College of Physicians of the United Kingdom
MRCS**	Member of the Royal College of Surgeons
FRCAnaes	Fellow of the Royal College of Anaesthetists
FRCR	Fellow of the Royal College of Radiologists
FRCOphth	Fellow of the Royal College of Ophthalmology
MRCOG*	Member of the Royal College of Obstetricians and Gynaecologists
MRCPsych*	Member of the Royal College of Psychiatrists
MRCPath*	Member of the Royal College of Pathologists
MRCGP***	Member of the Royal College of General Practitioners
MFPHM*	Member of the Faculty of Public Health Medicine of the Royal College of Physicians
MRCPCH*	Member of the Royal College of Paediatrics and Child Health

*Fellowship is by election after an interval of several years.
**Fellowship follows further higher exams and training.
***Fellowship can be by election or assessment.

The specialist register

Satisfactory completion of a programme of appropriate specialist training complying with the requirements of the European Medical Directive leads to a Certificate of Completion of Specialist Training (CCST), which confers specialist status throughout the European Union. The Specialist Training Authority (STA) of the Royal Colleges and the Joint Committee on Postgraduate Training for General Practice (JCPTGP) are statutorily responsible for certificating the satisfactory completion of training for entry to a specialty. In the United Kingdom the certificate then has to be registered with the GMC, which is responsible for keeping the specialist register. Each programme and rotation of training posts must be approved by the Royal College appropriate to the specialty. Specialists trained overseas who have had training equivalent to the CCST standards and doctors who have had a more research-based training but are considered to have CCST level still can be entered on the specialist register on recommendation of the STA without going through a standard programme. Since January 1997, being on the specialist register has been a legal requirement before a doctor may take up a consultant (specialist) appointment in the United Kingdom.

Appointments to the specialist registrar grade are made in open competition on a regional basis organised by the postgraduate dean in that region, apart from specialist training programmes in the armed forces for which special arrangements apply. On entry into a specialist training programme a doctor receives a national training number (NTN) which is retained throughout training even if part of the training is taken in approved research at home or in approved posts abroad. The number may also be retained for a limited time after acquisition of the CCST if the new specialist remains in a training post before obtaining a consultant appointment.

The training numbers act as a passport to education in that specialty, guaranteeing a continued training post subject to satisfactory progression.

Many specialist training programmes lead to a dual CCST, for example in general and vascular surgery or general medicine and gastroenterology. Having the general certification is important for those helping to provide the acute emergency intaking service. Few hospitals have so many specialists on the staff that they can afford the luxury of specialists who do not at the same time also have the ability to look after acute emergencies competently as part of their task. Very few doctors specialise solely in acute emergency medicine at present, not to be confused with accident and emergency (A & E) doctors who see patients in the accident and emergency department and then pass them on for admission and management by the duty specialist team, if necessary. Some accident and emergency consultants look after these patients for the first 24 hours in an observation ward from which they are then either discharged or admitted under a specialist team.

Overseas doctors without the right of indefinite residence or settled status in the United Kingdom or who do not benefit from European Union rights (regardless of where they obtained their medical qualification) may compete for a place on specialist training programmes which confer a fixed term training appointment (FTTA) and which are open only to overseas doctors. At present, these doctors may stay in the United Kingdom for only four years of postgraduate training. Such programmes do not lead to a CCST but the doctor is entitled to a certificate recording the specialist training undertaken.

Part time (flexible) training is possible for CCST. These programmes are aimed particularly but not exclusively at women doctors who wish to combine specialist training with family responsibilities, retaining their interests and skills in a specialist career. Doctors wishing to enter a specialist training programme as flexible trainees must satisfy the postgraduate dean that training on a full time basis would not be practicable. Full time trainees can apply to become flexible trainees and flexible trainees can apply to revert to full time training at any time. The United Kingdom health departments have required postgraduate deans to maximise flexible training opportunities. The total duration and quality of training must be not less than that required for full time trainees.

Before they even reach the stage of competing for a specialist registrar post many women doctors take advantage of the doctors' retainer scheme established to encourage those temporarily unable to practice because of domestic commitments to remain in touch with medical activity and continue their training to return eventually to substantial practice. They are expected to work up to a maximum of two paid sessions weekly in hospital or in general practice to a total of at least 12 sessions a year for which they receive in addition to their pay for these sessions an annual retainer which covers their subscription to the GMC (essential to maintain registration) and a subscription to a professional journal. They are also expected to attend at least seven educational sessions annually.

All specialties have specialist registrar training schemes designed essentially for doctors who will become consultants or general practitioners in the NHS. A much smaller parallel stream of clinical lecturer/honorary specialist registrar combines NHS clinical experience in a university teaching hospital with a much larger research and teaching opportunity. As the CCST requires a strongly service-based training to ensure high standards of clinical practice, those proceeding through the academic route will usually take longer to obtain their certificate. Their training may also be prolonged by two or three years for whole time study leading to a PhD, awarded for a thesis based on laboratory research, but this is often completed before they start specialist clinical training.

Consultants

After obtaining the CCST, doctors compete for a consultant post. Insofar that the term implies giving advice rather than hands-on examination and treatment as part of a team, the term is outdated and misleading. Senior doctors with full responsibility would more precisely be described as specialists, whether in hospital, general practice, or public health. There would be logic in progressing from specialist registrar to specialist, rather than to consultant, but the profession is not always governed by logic. Doubtless it will come eventually and no one will then understand why there was ever a problem.

Currently, the relationship between consultant vacancies and the number of specialist registrars nearing the end of their training differs greatly between specialties. In most specialties newly qualified specialists have no difficulty in finding a consultant job, particularly if they are prepared to move to another part of the country. Doctors who have taken their specialist training in academic units often continue in university hospitals either as senior lecturers with honorary consultant status or as NHS consultants, some become NHS consultants in district general hospitals, and a few go into clinical research or management in the pharmaceutical industry. Senior lecturers may be promoted in due course to reader or professor.

The NHS does not have different levels of seniority of consultant but it does reward exceptional service and scientific distinction with distinction awards, salary supplements which at the highest level are substantial in relation to the basic salary. Not all doctors in the hospital service aspire to become consultants; they may become an associate specialist, part time medical officer (clinical assistant), hospital practitioner, or staff doctor, a grade established for those who have not completed a formal specialist training programme or do not wish to have the full range of responsibilities of a consultant. These posts are advertised nationally in the same way as all other medical posts in the NHS, with the exception of preregistration house officer posts linked with particular medical schools which are filled internally.

Consultants may undertake private practice alongside their NHS responsibilities. If their earnings from private practice exceed more than 10% of their NHS salary, they must give up part of their NHS salary. Their status as a specialist in private practice is underwritten by the fact that they have obtained a consultant post in open competition after a full period of rigorous training. A curious and peculiarly English myth has long promoted the public belief that solely private practitioners in Harley Street are the best. The reverse is likely to be true because most practitioners who do not also work as consultants in the NHS have not completed an accredited specialist training or, if they have, have not obtained a consultant post in open competition, with the exception of a few who have already been NHS consultants and have given up their public service to work solely in private practice. There is nothing to stop any doctor fully registered with the GMC from setting up as a private specialist, but in future doctors not listed on the *specialist register* will not be eligible for payment as a specialist through insurance schemes. They may also find it difficult to satisfy Royal College's expectations that they are regularly keeping up to date in their relatively isolated position.

Appraisal and revalidation

Whatever the specialty, all registered medical practitioners will in future be regularly appraised in the context of their work to ensure that they are maintaining satisfactory standards. This has become the norm in other professions and there is no reason for doctors to be an exception, except that it has been difficult to devise an appropriate and efficient way of undertaking appraisal in clinical specialties without creating a whole new work agenda for very busy people.

Every five years, the portfolio of a doctor's appraisals will be submitted as evidence for revalidation of registration with the GMC. Again, there is a formidable need to devise a system which is practical, cost effective, and sufficient to maintain confidence in the profession.

REMEMBER

- Medicine offers secure, relatively well paid employment in a large variety of possible careers.

- Students should start to consider their career options by their fourth or fifth year at medical school. Many have no firm intentions at this stage beyond knowing a few areas which they have discounted.

- Most doctors choose their specialty towards the end of their house officer year but around a third will change their mind over the next three years, sometimes more than once. The commonest reason for changing choice is personal and family commitments.

- Specialties vary substantially in the amount of emergency work, and therefore in the disruption of personal life.

- "Flexible" part time training is possible in most specialties for those for whom full time training is not practicable.

- Some specialties are more popular than others, and this is ever-changing. It pays to explore all the options.

- Some doctors are able to combine more than one specialty, such as general practice and a clinical assistantship in a hospital discipline or public health or medical journalism.

- All doctors in the NHS—whether consultants or principles in general practice—need to obtain a Certificate of Completion of Specialist Training or Certificate of Prescribed Training in General Practice.

- An increasing number of junior doctors spend time out of the NHS, travelling, working abroad, working in a different field or just taking out a gap year. For most this gives them time to settle on their intended career options and keep a healthy perspective on their life, and it is no longer regarded unfavourably by many employers.

- In future all doctors, whatever their chosen specialty, will have to undergo a system of appraisal of their knowledge and skills every five years, which will be compulsory for revalidation of their GMC registration.

12. Career opportunities

Medicine offers an amazing range of different career options. Most doctors end up in general practice, hospital specialties, or public health. Medical students are well advised to take a careful look at the very broad canvas of opportunity before they qualify. Most people finally choose their specialty within two or three years of graduation. However an increasing number of doctors choose careers which are more varied, include other interests, and are flexible enough to allow them to fit their career around their life, not the other way round.

General practice (Figure 12.1)

To become a principal in general practice, a doctor must complete three years' vocational training. This includes at least 12 months as a GP registrar; two periods of at least six months each in educationally approved training posts drawn from a list of hospital specialties particularly relevant to general practice, such as paediatrics, care of the elderly, obstetrics and gynaecology, psychiatry, and accident and emergency; and the remainder of the time in hospital or community medicine. Any or all of the training may be undertaken part time provided the whole process is completed within seven years. Training is carefully and continuously supervised by specially trained and accredited general practitioners, who guide and monitor training through a process of summative assessment. This assessment includes written examinations, discussion of videos of their own consultations, an audit project, and a report from the trainer; experience is recorded in a log book. Successful completion of the training is marked by the award of a Certificate of Prescribed Experience in General Practice issued by the Joint Committee on Postgraduate General Practice Training.

	Optional	Vocational training		
Preregistration house officer →	Senior house officer →	Senior house officer →	General practice reg →	General practice principal →
Medicine/surgery	Any specialty	Relevant specialties	General practice	General practice
1 year	1–2 years	2 years	1 year	Career post

Figure 12.1—Structure of training for a career in general practice.

General practitioners are still in short supply in some parts of the country and most new GPs eventually join a partnership of established GPs. However an increasing number of newly qualified GPs work in a variety of shorter term jobs for several years before committing to joining a practice. A growing number of salaried GP posts exist, some combining general practice with teaching or research, or work in a different clinical field such as accident and emergency or a medical specialty outpatient clinic. Job vacancies of all types are advertised in the medical press, such as the *BMJ*, and are filled in open competition.

General practice (family medicine) is a demanding but fulfilling career. As a new GP you can choose how many sessions you wish to work each week which allows you greater flexibility to combine being a GP with outside interests such as raising a family or developing skills in research or another clinical area in a hospital clinical assistant post. It offers the prospect of a settled home and higher income at an earlier stage than a career in the hospital service. General practitioners who live (as most do) in the district in which they practise, naturally become very much part of their local community and have the satisfaction of giving long term continuity of care, unless practising in an inner city where the population is continuously changing and where as many as a third of the general practitioner's patients may change each year. GPs are taking on an increasing role in the planning of all hospital and community services through Primary Care Trusts which are changing the way GPs work all across the country.

After completing a three year training scheme, or after being fully registered for four years of which two have been spent in general practice, a doctor may take the examination for membership of the Royal College of General Practitioners (MRCGP) but it is not an essential qualification. There are also a number of other postgraduate diplomas which can be taken, such as the DCH (Diploma in Child Health) and the DRCOG (Diploma of the Royal College of Obstetricians and Gynaecologists). An increasing number of GPs study for a Masters Degree; a few undertake research for an MD. The only essential qualification is a Certificate of Prescribed Experience in General Practice.

Hospital specialties (Figure 12.2)

The broad structure of specialist training leading to the Certificate of Completion of Specialist Training (CCST) is similar in all hospital specialties. From qualification to recognition as a specialist normally takes about seven years: the final year of basic medical education and training (the preregistration house officer year), about two years general professional training (at senior house officer level), and a four year specialist registrar programme. Specialties such as cardiology and cardiac surgery, which are particularly dependent on practical skill, take the longest.

Accident and emergency

People with acute injuries or sudden acute illness often dial 999 for the ambulance service, are picked up from the street, or are urgently sent to hospital by their doctor. Others taken less acutely or seriously ill, who for one reason or another do not want to or cannot call their general practitioner, take themselves straight to hospital. Many accident and emergency departments include both a minor injuries unit run entirely by nurse practitioners and the consultant led medical team who provide for the patients requiring acute resuscitation, full medical assessment, or more complicated medical treatment. The consultants are in overall charge of the whole team, but the initial sorting of cases is the responsibility of an experienced nurse who also ensures appropriate destination and priority for each individual.

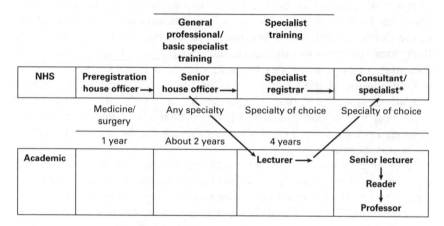

		General professional/ basic specialist training	Specialist training	
NHS	**Preregistration house officer →**	**Senior house officer →**	**Specialist registrar →**	**Consultant/ specialist***
	Medicine/ surgery	Any specialty	Specialty of choice	Specialty of choice
	1 year	About 2 years	4 years	
Academic			**Lecturer →**	**Senior lecturer** ↓ **Reader** ↓ **Professor**

Figure 12.2—Structure of training for a hospital specialty in either the NHS or clinical academic (university) posts.

*Some specialists choose not to take on consultants' responsibilities such as out of hours on call and work as Associate Specialists or Staff Grade Specialists. These are often part time and less well paid than consultants.

Dealing with anything and everything serious, not so serious, or difficult to discern requires special skill, training, and experience, useful whatever medical specialty a doctor eventually ends up in. For that reason, many senior house officer training programmes in medicine, surgery, and several other specialties now include a period of several months in the accident and emergency department to develop this core dimension of practical professional skill. Telling the difference between the apparently trivial and a medical or surgical time bomb is an art fully learnt only through active service in front line trenches; getting it right, or at least not sending the patient home without fail safe follow up, can save tens of lives and hundreds of thousands of pounds in medical litigation fees and damages.

Accident and emergency consultants have in the past usually had a background in surgery, medicine, anaesthetics, or general practice. Specific training programmes now exist leading to becoming a Fellow of the Faculty of Accident and Emergency Medicine (FFAEM). Accident and emergency is one of the few clinical specialties which readily lends itself to shift working. Most patients are treated and referred back to their GPs so there is little call for continuity of care. Learning from experience is assured by regular meetings of the whole team to review successes and failures.

Anaesthetics

Anaesthetics is another specialty in which continuity of care is limited: preoperative assessment, the operation itself, the early recovery period, and intermittent periods of responsibility for supervising the intensive care unit. It is a very hands on specialty and if you are up all night provision is normally made for you to be off for at least part of the next day. The work of an anaesthetist falls fairly tidily into regular and carefully defined commitments.

Providing pain relief or anaesthesia during surgical operations, childbirth, and diagnostic procedures is the major task of an anaesthetist. Most also take turns in charge of the intensive care unit and an increasing number confine themselves to such work. Anaesthetics is a large and expanding specialty.

The primary examination for Fellowship of the Royal College of Anaesthetists (FRCAnaes) can be taken 18 months after graduation, usually taken during a senior house officer post in anaesthetics, and is a test of knowledge of the scientific basis of anaesthetics and anaesthesia. The final part of the FRCAnaes is taken after one year as a specialist registrar.

Medicine

Specialists in medicine in the United Kingdom are known as "physicians". On the whole, medicine and surgery attract different personalities: physicians tend to be more reflective; surgeons more executive. The difference is reflected in the respective Royal Colleges as Dr John Rowan Wilson observed some years ago but nothing much has changed:

> The Royal Colleges are, of course, much the smarter end of the profession; they represent the big time. However, the two main colleges, the Physicians, and the Surgeons, are very different in character. The Royal College of Physicians, like the Catholic Church, is ancient and obscurely hierarchical. It occupies a tiny Vatican in Regents Park, whose benign soft-footed cardinals pad around discussing preferment of one kind or another. To be a Member of the College (achieved by examination) counts for nothing at all. One must be elected a Fellow. ... In turning to the College of Surgeons one moves from the episcopal to the military. Surgeons are brash, extrovert characters who pride themselves on energy rather than subtlety. Fellowship is decided by examination, and theoretically all Fellows are equal, just as theoretically all officers are gentlemen.

121

Some physicians are narrow subspecialists in a subject such as dermatology (skin diseases) or rheumatology (joint and muscle disorders) but most have dual certification in general medicine and a subspecialty. "Internal" is sometimes added to the title of general medicine because that is the North American term for the specialty.

The "general" label, means that the physician can successfully bat any acute medical emergency balls—at least hitting them towards an appropriate fielder. In practice, this requires the ability to cope with any and every acute medical emergency, at least in the initial stage, and the ability to deal with unstructured diagnostic problems not falling obviously into any particular subspecialty at an early stage. Most British hospitals are not large enough either to have a specialist in each subspecialty of medicine or to maintain an acute medical emergency rota for patients who need to be admitted to hospital at any hour of the day or night without the participation of most of the specialist physicians. The position is similar in surgery.

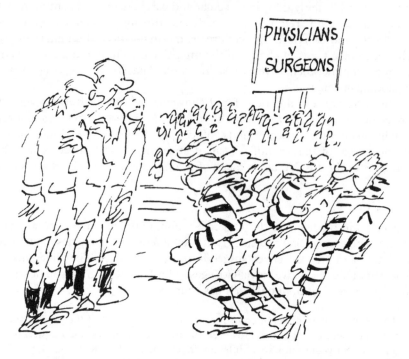

Time and again, hospital specialist practice requires well informed clinical common sense rather than intensely specialised knowledge. Professor J R A Mitchell told the story of a patient who reappeared in his outpatient clinic, having being referred from specialist to specialist, saying, "there is no point in sending me to another specialist, doctor, it is not my special parts which have gone wrong but what holds them together".

Membership of the Royal Colleges of Physicians of the United Kingdom (MRCP (UK)) is the professional diploma needed before you embark on specialist training in any of the specialties listed under medicine in Table 12.1. The Royal Colleges of Physicians in London and Edinburgh and the Royal College of Physicians and Surgeons in Glasgow hold a common membership examination. Election to fellowship normally follows about 10 years after passing the examination for membership.

The MRCP diploma is a necessary entry qualification but confers no right to a training number in a medical specialty. Although the examination is difficult and the pass rate low, more doctors are successful in the examination than can become specialists in medicine. Some deliberately acquire the diploma as an additional qualification before entering another hospital specialty or general practice. Part I of the examination can be taken 18 months after graduation and comprises multiple choice questions covering a wide range of medicine and the sciences immediately relevant to it. Part II can be taken after one year in approved posts providing experience of responsibility for acute general medical emergencies and consists of a written section, including questions on interpretation of case histories and slides, and a searching clinical examination. The clinical and oral examinations were previously taken either in adult medicine or paediatrics but there is now a separate diploma of MRCPCH—Membership of the Royal College of Paediatrics and Child Health (see below).

The MRCP examination is, above all, a test of clinical skills: it covers similar ground to the final MB examination in medicine but at a more demanding and discriminating level. It is necessary to know about rarities but it is even more important to have sound clinical skill and common sense, based on expertise in managing everyday medical emergencies.

Paediatrics and child health

The care of children, especially of the newborn, has become immensely specialised. Forty years ago, paediatrics was part of general medicine, but not now. The skills required are very different from those required in adult medicine and so too is the spectrum of disease. Until recently, the specialist qualification for entry to paediatrics was the MRCP(UK), which could be taken specifically in paediatrics as well as in adult medicine. The special nature of paediatrics, its role and range across the divide between hospital and community and the interplay of medical, psychiatric, and social factors in child care was finally and formally recognised by the founding of the Royal College of Paediatrics and Child Health in 1996, which has developed its own membership examination.

Paediatric subspecialties are less well developed than those in adult medicine and practically all paediatricians working at any but the very largest and most specialised hospitals need to participate also in a general emergency service, either in neonatal intensive care, acute paediatrics, or child protection. Paediatrics is a specialty in which consultants have a particularly large personal hands on involvement in the acute emergency work. Specialist training is likewise very practically intensive. Children

123

Nov. 2003 (handwritten)

Table 12.1—Major specialties and their required professional higher qualifications

Specialty	Qualification
General practice	MRCGP*
Hospital specialties	
Accident and emergency	FFAEM
Anaesthesia	FRCAnaes
Medicine	MRCP
General (internal) medicine	
Cardiology	
Clinical immunology (see also pathology)	
Clinical pharmacology	
Communicable (infectious) diseases	
Dermatology	
Endocrinology and diabetes	
Genitourinary medicine (venereology)	
Care of the elderly	
Haematology (see also pathology)	
Metabolic medicine	
Neurology	
Oncology (see also radiotherapy)	
Renal disease (nephrology)	
Respiratory disease	
Rheumatology	
Tropical medicine	
Obstetrics and gynaecology	MRCOG
Ophthalmology	FRCOphth
Pathology	MRCPath
Clinical biochemistry	
Haematology	
Blood transfusion	
Histopathology	
Immunopathology	
Medical microbiology	
Forensic pathology	
Clinical immunology	
Paediatrics	MRCPCH
Psychiatry	MRCPsych
Adult psychiatry	
Child psychiatry	
Forensic psychiatry	
Mental handicap	
Psychogeriatrics	
Psychotherapy	
Diagnostic radiology	FRCR
Radiotherapy and oncology	FRCR (MRCP)
Rehabilitation	MRCP, FRCS
Surgery	MRCS/FRCS
General surgery	
Neurosurgery	
Orthopaedics	
Otorhinolaryngology (ENT)	
Paediatric surgery	
Plastic surgery	
Urology	
Public health medicine	MFPHM
Other specialties	
Occupational medicine	MRCP, MFOM
Armed services	
Pharmaceutical industry	
Full time research	
Basic medical sciences	
Medical journalism	

*MRCGP is not essential for entry to general practice.

Handwritten annotations:
- (3 yrs.) → General practice
- (7 yrs. or more) → Medicine
- Anaesthesia (go for family, shifts = bad, v. chemistry orientated)
- Ophthalmology (not as gory, short operations)
- Paediatrics (bad shifts) for having family
- Psychiatry — for having family
- Radiotherapy and oncology (includes lots of physics)
- Neurosurgery (10 hr. long surgery – mainly men do)
- (3 yrs. including pre-reg. yr.) → Surgery / General surgery

become seriously ill very quickly and, with immediate intervention, can improve just as fast. More and more hospital based paediatrics is spreading out into the care of children in the community, an aspect of the specialty given the American style name of "ambulatory" paediatrics.

Obstetrics and gynaecology

Obstetrics and gynaecology is one specialty with two different aspects. Obstetrics offers a balance between medicine and surgery with the attraction of usually young and healthy patients and a happy outcome to the encounter. Gynaecology (diseases specifically of women) also demands both surgical and medical skills.

Specialists in this field become members of the Royal College of Obstetricians and Gynaecologists (MRCOG). Part I of the examination, a multiple choice paper on the basic sciences, is related to the specialty and may be taken at any time after full registration. Part II is taken after at least three years in approved posts and includes written, clinical, and oral examinations, together with preparation of case records and commentaries. Instruction in family planning is included in the training. Some obstetricians train first in general surgery and obtain the Fellowship of a Royal College of Surgeons (FRCS) to acquire a much wider surgical ability than their limited surgical specialty necessarily demands; a few start in medicine (particularly endocrinology) and first pass the MRCP; an occasional brilliant workhorse obtains both these diplomas and the MRCOG.

Pathology

The specialties within pathology provide a wide range of laboratory diagnostic services which are an essential part of everyday clinical practice. The clinical biochemist is an expert in the biochemical mechanisms and diagnosis of disease; the histopathologist and cytologist is an expert in diagnosing disease from changes in tissue or cell structure; and the medical microbiologist (a title which includes bacteriologist, virologist, and mycologist) is an expert in the culture and identification of bacteria, viruses, fungi, and other communicable causes of disease. Some medical microbiologists combine this diagnostic function with the detection, epidemiological monitoring, and control of outbreaks of infection, based in one of the laboratories of the Public Health Laboratory Service.

The haematologist is concerned with disorders of the blood and with blood transfusion; some haematologists specialise entirely in blood transfusion and work for the National Blood Transfusion Service. Clinical immunology is a small but expanding specialty which spans laboratory science and clinical medicine. It is concerned particularly with the role of immune reactions in disease. Although based in the laboratory, pathologists often consult on patients at their colleagues' request. The medical microbiologist for example should be in a position to give expert advice on antibiotic treatment of serious infections and on the control of the spread of infections in hospital.

Haematologists normally have patients under their care in wards and outpatients. Besides having scientific and clinical skills, the consultant pathologist needs to be capable of becoming a good director of a laboratory.

For a career in all these pathology specialties, with the exception of clinical immunology for which the MRCP may be more appropriate and haematology for which it is customary to have both memberships, it is necessary to become a member of the Royal College of Pathologists (MRC Path). The part I examination is taken after three years in one of the many specialties of pathology. It is no longer a test of all branches of pathology. Part II is taken at a minimum of two years after part I and is limited to the chosen specialty. Unlike the MRCP, which is in effect an entry qualification to specialisation in medicine, acquisition of the MRC Path marks the completion of training as a pathologist. The FRC Path is granted about 12 years later.

Psychiatry

Psychiatry is an expanding specialty which is changing rapidly, not least because new treatments are substantially reducing the need for inpatient treatment, especially the need for long stay mental hospitals. Political policy has also moved many long term psychiatric patients out of hospital into a community which unfortunately cannot always cope with them or they with the community. Psychiatry includes the subspecialty of mental handicap, a Cinderella subject with the task of deploying a range of medical and engineering skills, together with human insight to help handicapped patients realise their own potential. The emphasis in their care is shifting towards rehabilitation in small units before they attempt to return to their own homes.

The examination for membership of the Royal College of Psychiatrists (MRC Psych) may be taken after three years of approved experience, most of which has to be in psychiatry. This means working as a specialist registrar in a psychiatric hospital looking after both emergency and long stay patients, besides seeing patients in the psychiatric outpatient clinic. It is possible to specialise in either adult or child psychiatry but all psychiatrists are expected to have some experience of both.

A good knowledge of medicine is valuable in psychiatry, and some psychiatrists acquire the MRCP in the early years of their training.

Diagnostic radiology

Like pathologists, radiologists need to be good organisers because sooner or later they are likely to have to manage all or part of a department. They need to be skilled with their hands in performing invasive investigations, such as cannulation of internal vessels and biopsy of deep seated lumps under screening, and in interventional techniques, such as angioplasty (dilatation of narrow blood vessels). They also need to be sharp with their eyes and quick with their brains in interpreting x ray films and scans. Responsibility for radioisotope investigations normally also falls within the responsibility of the radiologist. Many radiologists obtain the MRCP or occasionally the FRCS while gaining clinical experience before taking up radiology. Diagnostic radiology serves all clinical departments and often provides an open access service for general practitioners as well. Advances in radiology, particularly computerised scanning, have transformed clinical practice in many specialties. Radiologists therefore have a natural link with most of their colleagues. They also have contact with patients but without overall clinical responsibility for their treatment. Out of hours duties are generally not heavy with the exception of subspecialties such as neuroradiology.

Fellowship of the Royal College of Radiologists (FRCR) is a necessary qualification. Part I is taken after at least one year in a recognised specialist training post and part II after at least three years of training.

Radiotherapy and oncology

Cancer is treated by radiotherapy, drugs, and surgery. Treatment of cancer by irradiation (radiotherapy) or by drugs (chemotherapy) falls to different specialists: the clinical oncologist (previously called radiotherapist) and the medical oncologist, respectively. They undertake overlapping but partly different training, leading to the FRCR (and may also obtain the MRCP). Successful treatment of cancer requires teamwork, and clinical oncologists and medical oncologists not only work closely with each other but also with other specialties, especially with surgeons, physicians, and gynaecologists.

Part I of the FRCR examination is common to diagnostic radiology and radiotherapy, but they have a different part II examination.

Rehabilitation

Rehabilitation is concerned with the active and optimistic management of disability, both acute after stroke or serious injury and chronic disability. The specialty requires the ability to encourage, motivate, and inspire both clients and their families. The ability to earn the respect of a multidisciplinary team of doctors, nurses, physiotherapists, and social workers is invaluable. It is useful to be good with your hands, and to have an understanding of the potential of both electrical and mechanical engineering as well as computer science. A professional background in neurology or orthopaedics may be particularly appropriate but above all the specialty requires humanity, perseverance, realistic optimism, and boundless energy.

Surgery

Surgery was once considered a craft rather than as a now well established intellectual and practical art. Surgical specialties are, in a manner of speaking, more cut and dried than medical specialties, as Henri de Mondeville observed in the 13th century:

> Surgery is superior to Medicine, because among other things it is more lucrative. To receive gifts or money, a surgeon dare not fear stench, must be able to cut like an executioner, politely lie and be clever. ... The sick above all want to be cured; the surgeon to be paid.

Surgical training is divided into two parts: basic surgical training applicable to all surgical specialties and subspecialty training. Surgeons often obtain dual certification in general surgery and a subspecialty because most consultant surgeons are expected to cover acute surgical emergencies and undertake some relatively unspecialised surgery besides having a special field of expertise.

Basic surgical training follows preregistration house officer appointments with about two years in the senior house officer grade. At the end of that time the trainee should have sufficient knowledge and skills to pursue career training in surgery as a specialist registrar. Basic training includes study of the basic medical sciences, together with experience in general surgery, accident and emergency, and orthopaedic surgery. The MRCS examination is taken at the end of this period.

The trainee then competes for a surgical specialist registrar post, which provides training in both general surgery and a subspecialty, except for those who concentrate entirely on becoming ear, nose, and throat (ENT) or eye (ophthalmic) surgeons. There are seven recognised surgical subspecialties at present (see Table 12.1, p. 124). Towards the end of this period of surgical specialist training there is a further examination, the FRCS, which is an examination run by the four surgical colleges of Great Britain and Ireland. The examination particularly tests clinical skills and, together with the necessary years of experience, qualifies the trainee for the CCST.

Public health medicine

Public health is the medical specialty which is concerned with the improvement of the health of populations—by health promotion and disease prevention and by commissioning high quality, cost effective health care from providers of health care, mainly hospitals and general practitioners. Public health doctors work closely with doctors in many specialties and with other health professionals, with managers, and with governmental and voluntary organisations. Public health recognises that health requires more than individual patient care. If all members of society are to achieve a better and more equitable health status and health experience, collective action is essential.

It is worth remembering that public health doctors have had every bit as great, if not greater, impact on improving health than physicians and surgeons. A tablet to William Henry Duncan, Medical Officer of Health of Liverpool, who died in 1863, records that "... under the blessing of God he succeeded in reducing the rate of mortality in Liverpool by nearly one third". Epidemiology, the discipline concerned with describing and explaining the occurrence of disease in populations (originally epidemics of infectious disease) and of the outcome of measures to improve health and prevent disease, is the science fundamental to public health medicine and indeed to a substantial proportion of modern medical research. Public health doctors also require a range of other skills, most crucially those associated with management, interpersonal, and political skills in representing the need for more resources for health care and for better use of them.

Public health physicians work in a number of settings within the NHS, the university, central government, and national agencies, such as the Health Education Authority and the Communicable Diseases Surveillance Centre (which is part of the Public Health Laboratory Service (PHLS)).

Two years of general professional and early specialist training culminate in part I of the examination for membership of the Faculty of Public Health Medicine (MFPHM of the Royal College of Physicians of London), which covers epidemiology, statistics, social and behavioural sciences, the principles of prevention of disease and promotion of health, assessment of health needs and audit of services provided, environmental health, and the management and organisation of health services. It is a rapidly expanding specialty. During three years of higher specialist training, the trainee in public health medicine writes a report on practical projects as part of the requirement for part II of the MFPHM examination.

Community health

Doctors working in community health are clinical specialists providing a wide range of services, including child health; family planning; mental and physical handicap; genetic counselling; occupational, environmental, and port health; and community services for the elderly. A relevant clinical specialist training or general practitioner vocational training is the usual qualification for this work, but there are, as yet, no formal relevant community higher specialist training programmes or qualifications.

Most of the doctors are in the grades of clinical medical officer (CMO) and senior clinical medical officer (SCMO). A small but increasing number of consultant posts have been established in these community specialties and training programmes for such posts are being developed.

Other specialties

Clinical academic medicine

A degree of creative tension often exists between the NHS consultants and clinical academic (university) staff, well expressed by the Royal Commission on Medical Education in 1968:

> There are still full-time academic teachers who see the part-timer as a prosperous busy practitioner who owes his success to clinical acumen rather than painstaking investigation, whose teaching is based on personal dogma

rather than scientific fact and whose interests require the whims of private patients to take priority over the needs of his students. There are still part-time teachers who see the full-timer as a desiccated preacher more interested in the advancement of medicine than in the welfare of his patients and unable to offer his students any guidance to the realities of life outside the ivory tower.

There is a smattering of truth in each perspective to the extent that the clinical academic physician or surgeon was described by Dean Holly Smith as "an uneasy hybrid who constantly feels attenuated at both ends".

An academic career in university posts is possible in practically all hospital specialties, general practice, and public health, though the number of posts is small. Clinical senior lecturers, readers, and professors all normally have NHS consultant responsibilities, but they generally have less clinical service work and relatively more time than NHS consultants for teaching and research.

Basic medical sciences

It is widely but not universally believed that medical students benefit from being taught anatomy, physiology, biochemistry, and pharmacology by medical graduates because they best understand the clinical context of these sciences and their relevance to clinical medicine. Few medical graduates, however, now work in these university departments, not least because salaries are lower than those of clinical academics and of other doctors working in the NHS.

Full time research

A small number of full time research posts are available to medical graduates, mainly in institutions of the Medical Research Council or in the pharmaceutical industry.

Occupational medicine

Doctors have long been involved in the understanding and preventing of health risks in the workplace but only recently has occupational medicine developed as a clinical specialty rather than as a branch of public health. It includes the former discipline of industrial medicine. The specialty is concerned with identifying and investigating the medical problems associated with different working environments and with advising both management and employees on the prevention of occupational medical hazards.

The examination for membership of the Faculty of Occupational Medicine (MFOM) of the Royal College of Physicians of London is taken after four years of training and experience in occupational medicine; a formal higher specialist training programme leads up to it. Occupational medicine is another specialty suitable for part time service.

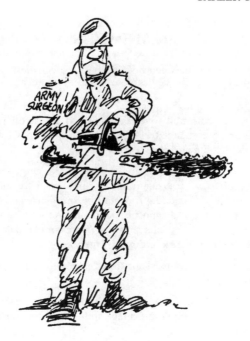

Armed services

The three major branches of the armed services offer careers for both hospital specialists and general practitioners on long or short term contracts. Many doctors begin a service career with a short service commission while they are medical students. In return for a good salary during clinical training and the preregistration year these doctors are required to serve for a further five years in the armed services.

Pharmaceutical industry

The pharmaceutical industry employs an increasing number of doctors in clinical research and in an advisory capacity. Most doctors entering the industry have a good background in clinical pharmacology or specialist medicine.

Medical journalism

The *BMJ*, the *Lancet*, and a number of other publications have full time medically qualified editors, together with some who are not medically qualified. Many specialist medical journals have part time medical editors, as do several newspapers and industrially sponsored medical publications. Freelance opportunities in journalism, radio, and television abound for fluent doctors with lively minds, even if they are not Jonathan Millers. You might even become a novelist or playwright along with Somerset Maugham, Chekhov, and many others by dipping your creative pen into your medical life experience.

131

REMEMBER

- The broad choice is between hospital-based specialties, general practice or public health.

- General practice allows greater continuity of care of families and individuals in a community over a long period. It also offers more flexible working hours, the chance to be "more your own boss", a settled home and a higher income and at an earlier stage.

- The major hospital specialties are accident and emergency, anaesthesia, medical specialties (for example, cardiology, care of the elderly, gastroenterology, dermatology), obstetrics and gynaecology, paediatrics, psychiatry, pathology, diagnostic radiology, radiotherapy and cancer, ophthalmology, and surgical specialties (for example, colorectal surgery, orthopaedic surgery, ear/nose/throat surgery).

- Increasing opportunities exist for non-consultant senior grades in some hospital specialties.

- Public health medicine is concerned with the improvement of the health of populations rather than individuals, and with the organisation of health service provision.

- Clinical academic medicine combines specialist training with enhanced opportunities for teaching and research.

- A few doctors follow careers in a variety of other fields, for example, the armed forces, occupational medicine, the pharmaceutical industry, or the media.

Postscript

On the decision to become a doctor rests the whole design and course of your life.

Being a doctor is something of a love–hate relationship. A recent graduate, who had had more than her fair share of difficulties as a student, described the feeling like this: "I am now working in a friendly district general hospital and I love it. I love being a doctor—at least I hate some of it but I am glad I went through medical school, resits and all."

We too are glad to be doctors, one up and coming, the other here and going. We have had our doubts: one of us seriously considered a career on the stage, the other as a historian (no prizes for guessing who was which). These remain our hobbies, unlike the famous cricketer, WG Grace, who took 10 years to qualify as a doctor, saying: "Medicine is my hobby, cricket is my profession." Those days are past.

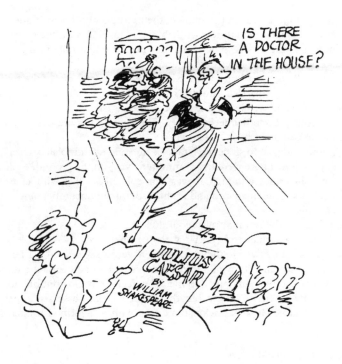

We cannot say what is right for you. We can only hope that we will have helped you towards your own well thought out decision. If you do decide that medicine is the career for you and are successful in gaining a place at medical school, we hope that this book will be your friend, guide, and encouragement throughout your student days.

For the last words we turn first to Susan Spindler, original producer of the BBC documentary series *Doctors to Be*, who once thought of becoming a doctor but decided against:

> Having observed hundreds of students and doctors over the past decade, I have a check list of qualities I look for in my doctors. I should like you to be kind, clever, and competent. I want you to know your way around the system, both in hospital and in the community. I hope you will like and will empathise with your patients wherever humanly possible and fight to give them the best treatment. And I'd like to think that you'll have managed to hang on to some of the ideals which drew you to medicine in the first place.

And finally, to Dr Farhad Islam, who as a student contributed his impressions of his first delivery (p. 80) and recently showed so graphically in an article reproduced here by courtesy of the *British Medical Journal*, how the years of learning medicine come together to make a competent and humane doctor, not forgetting in a moment of drama the need to be the patient's friend:

This time it was not a drill*

The phone rang. It was ten past nine in the morning and I wasn't due to start work in the casualty department at St Mary's Hospital until the afternoon.

"Where are you? It's Dad here. There's been a major rail crash just down the road from you. Hundreds are injured."

I quickly changed and ran downstairs. I weaved in and out of the traffic on my bicycle, and within two minutes I was at the police cordon. I flashed my identity badge and was led to the scene of the disaster.

"Keep your bicycle helmet on, Doc. The paramedics are over there with some of the wounded."

One hour had passed since the fatal collision and already a slick rescue plan was in operation. There were five commuters lying on the ground, each white with fear, shivering, although it was not cold. They lay with charred or bloodied faces. Looking dazed and frightened, but all uncomplaining—happy just to be alive.

I approached the trauma triage coordinator.

"Hello, I'm a casualty officer. How can I help?"

I was directed to two wounded passengers yet to see a doctor. I felt as if I was on autopilot, driven by all the procedures that I had been taught and all the duty that had been ingrained in me. That feeling would continue for most of the day. Basics first—airway, breathing, circulation. I assessed a man with a blackened face. He was obviously in pain with a deformed broken lower

---

*Taken from *BMJ* 1999;**319**:1079.

right leg. A paramedic was squeezing a bag of fluid into his veins to prevent shock. It was soon emptied and we had to wait for the next fleet of ambulances for more bags. He was stabilised and put into an ambulance, all the while thanking those around him.

I caught sight of a woman on the ground being comforted by a friend. She was visibly shaking. I peered into a large gash in her forehead. We immobilised her spine and put her in an ambulance.

The coordinator told me that it was unlikely that anyone else would be brought out alive from the wreckage. It was time to go to Mary's now. I grabbed my bike and sped down the main road still feeling as if some kind of compelling force was driving me. The whole experience was just so surreal. I had read the major incident plan two years before and remember being impressed by the precision and detail. There would be a press room; one room would be set up as a mortuary. I was reminded of the mock simulations of major incidents in my student days. Then volunteer students had been daubed in make up blood to act as casualties.

The accident and emergency department was a hive of activity. What struck me was that there seemed to be order, there seemed to be a plan—and it was working. It quickly dawned on me why I had not been rung. Doctors from all departments and specialties had rushed to help.

I was allotted a patient to look after and immediately recognised her as the woman I had attended at the scene. Now, like all the other patients, she had a number and I would be responsible for her. Around every patient was a dedicated team of doctor plus nurse.

Never had I imagined a major incident running so efficiently, especially with the horrific severity of injuries. The major incident packs, used for the first time, had all the necessary forms. Medical students stood ready to rush blood samples to the laboratories. I glimpsed the sight of patients with major burns being whisked away for emergency surgery.

My duty was to stay with my patient to continually assess her condition, anticipate potential problems, investigate and repair her wounds and be her friend. She had a nasty head injury and remained pale and cold. My main concern after establishing that her airway, breathing, and circulation were stable was to recognise that she might have a skull fracture and underlying serious head injury. The appropriate monitoring and tests were done.

It is funny how little things impress on your mind—hearing about members of the public ringing to donate blood, the catering department sending down sandwiches and drinks for exhausted staff, the gratitude of patients. All the while I was with my team, other teams were treating their own patients. Some were dreadfully burned, others had fractured limbs, ruptured spleens, or head injuries. I stitched up my patient's wounds with the help of a medical student. The nurses dressed her other wounds and we transferred her to the adjoining ward.

Suddenly the department was quiet and then the debriefing—lots of emotion, satisfaction, and pride on all sides for the sheer professionalism shown not just by the medical and nursing staff but by the porters, receptionists, police, security, and caterers.

FI

Appendices

Appendix 1   The core outcomes of basic medical education

The principles of professional practice

The principles of professional practice set out in *Good Medical Practice* must form the basis of medical education.

- *Good clinical care.* Doctors must practise good standards of clinical care, practise within the limits of their competence, and make sure that patients are not put at unnecessary risk.
- *Maintaining good medical practice.* Doctors must keep up to date with developments in their field and maintain their skills.
- *Relationships with patients.* Doctors must develop and maintain successful relationship with their patients.
- *Working with colleagues.* Doctors must work effectively with their colleagues.
- *Teaching and training.* If doctors have teaching responsibilities, they must develop the skills, attitudes, and practices of a competent teacher.
- *Probity.* Doctors must be honest.
- *Health.* Doctors must not allow their own health or condition to put patients at risk.

The following curricular outcomes are based on these principles. They set out what is expected of graduates. All curricula must include curricular outcomes that are consistent with those set out below.

Outcomes

Graduates must be able to do the following.

Good clinical care

(a) Know about and understand the following.
   (i)   Our guidance on the principles of good medical practice and the standards of competence, care, and conduct expected of doctors in the UK.
   (ii) The environment in which medicine is practised in the UK.
   (iii) How errors can happen in practice and the principles of managing risks.

136

(b) Know about, understand, and be able to apply and integrate the clinical, basic, behavioural, and social sciences on which medical practice is based.

(c) Be able to perform clinical and practical skills safely.

(d) Demonstrate the following attitudes and behaviour.

    (i) Recognise personal and professional limits, and be willing to ask for help when necessary.

    (ii) Recognise the duty to protect patients by taking action if a colleague's health, performance, or conduct is putting patients at risk.

Maintaining good medical practice

(a) Be able to gain, assess, apply, and integrate new knowledge and have the ability to adapt to changing circumstances throughout their professional life.

(b) Be willing to take part in continuing professional development to make sure that they maintain high levels of clinical competence and knowledge.

(c) Understand the principles of audit and the importance of using the results of audit to improve practice.

(d) Be willing to respond constructively to the outcomes of appraisal, performance review, and assessment.

Relationships with patients

(a) Know about and understand the rights of patients.

(b) Be able to communicate effectively with individuals and groups.

(c) Demonstrate the following attitudes and behaviour.

    (i) Accept the moral and ethical responsibilities involved in providing care to individual patients and communities.

    (ii) Respect patients regardless of their lifestyle, culture, beliefs, race, colour, gender, sexuality, disability, age, or social or economic status.

    (iii) Respect the right of patients to be fully involved in decisions about their care, including the right to refuse treatment or to refuse to take part in teaching or research.

    (iv) Recognise their obligation to understand and deal with patients' healthcare needs by consulting them and, where appropriate, their relatives or carers.

Working with colleagues

(a) Know about, understand and respect the roles and expertise of other health and social care professionals.

(b) Be able to demonstrate effective teamworking and leadership skills.

(c) Be willing to lead when faced with uncertainty and change.

Teaching and training

(a) Be able to demonstrate appropriate teaching skills.
(b) Be willing to teach colleagues and to develop their own teaching skills.

Probity

Graduates must demonstrate honesty in all areas of their professional work.

Health

Graduates must be aware of the importance of their own health, and its effect on their ability to practise as a doctor.

From *Tomorrow's Doctors*, 2nd edition, GMC, 2002.

Appendix 2   The aims of the Preregistration House Officer (PRHO) year ("general clinical training")

- When universities grant a registrable degree, they are certifying that their graduates have attained the goals of undergraduate medical education, as set out in the GMC's Recommendations on Undergraduate Medical Education, *Tomorrow's Doctors*, and that they have demonstrated competence in their published list of procedures.
- General clinical training is an integral part of basic medical education. Many of its aims are similar to those for undergraduate education and for the later stages of professional training, since medical education is a continuum. General clinical training builds on the attitudes, skills and knowledge graduates have developed and should enable them, as new doctors, to:
  (a) appreciate the centrality to the consultation by developing their competence in history taking, clinical examination, and the selection and interpretation of diagnostic tests
  (b) develop competence at diagnosis, decision making, and the provision of treatment, including prescribing
  (c) keep accurate records
  (d) refine the skills needed for the technical and practical procedures which any doctor should be able to perform
  (e) communicate effectively, both orally and in writing, with those with whom their professional practice brings them in contact: patients, relatives, healthcare professionals, and people in the community
  (f) develop and maintain respect for the dignity, privacy, and rights of patients, and concern for their relatives
  (g) work in a team and accept the principles of collective responsibility

(h) be aware of their own limitations and ready to seek help when necessary

(i) develop their knowledge and understanding of disease processes, including their natural history, the role of occupation in disease, and the possibilities for rehabilitation

(j) deepen their awareness of legal and ethical issues

(k) apply the principles of professional confidentiality in everyday practice

(l) understand the principles of evidence-based medicine

(m) understand the relationship between primary and social care and hospital care

(n) recognise and use opportunities for disease prevention and health promotion

(o) understand and use informatics as a tool in medical practice

(p) understand the purpose and practice of audit, peer review, and appraisal

(q) recognise self-education and professional development as a lifelong process

(r) develop appropriate attitudes towards personal health and well-being

(s) manage time effectively

(t) make the best use of laboratory and other diagnostic services

(u) follow safe practices (as detailed in their employer's occupational health and safety policy), relating to chemical, biological, physical, and psychological hazards in the workplace.

From *The New Doctor—Recommendations on General Clinical Training*, General Medical Council, 1997.

Appendix 3   Guidance to doctors

Being registered with the General Medical Council gives you rights and privileges. In return you must meet the standards of competence, care and conduct set by the GMC.

The duties of a doctor registered with the General Medical Council

Patients must be able to trust doctors with their lives and wellbeing. To justify that trust, we as a profession have a duty to maintain a good standard of practice and care and to show respect for human life. In particular as a doctor you must:

- Make the care of your patient your first concern
- Treat every patient politely and considerately

- Respect patients' dignity and privacy
- Listen to patients and respect their views
- Give patients information in a way they can understand
- Respect the rights of patients to be fully involved in decisions about their care
- Keep your professional knowledge and skills up to date
- Recognise the limits of your professional competence
- Be honest and trustworthy
- Respect and protect confidential information
- Make sure that your personal beliefs do not prejudice your patients' care
- Act quickly to protect patients from risk if you have good reason to believe that you or a colleague may not be fit to practice
- Avoid abusing your position as a doctor
- Work with colleagues in the ways that best serve patients' interests.

In all these matters you must never discriminate unfairly against your patients or colleagues. And you must always be prepared to justify your actions to them.

From *Good Medical Practice—Guidance from the General Medical Council,* 2001.

Appendix 4 Suggestions for further reading

Getting into Medical School by Jim Burnett. Trotman, 7th edition, 2002.

Insiders Guide to Medical Schools by Ian Urmston, Debbie Cohen, Richard Partridge. BMJ Books, 4th edition, 2001.

So You Want To Be a Doctor? by David Hopkins. Kogan Page, 1998.

A Career in Medicine. Do You Have What It Takes? by Harvey White. Royal Society of Medicine Press Ltd, 2000.

So You Want To Be A Brain Surgeon? A Medical Careers Guide by Chris Ward, Simon Eccles. Oxford University Press, 2nd edition, 2001.

Getting Into Medicine: The Essential Guide To Choosing A Medical School And Obtaining A Place by Andrew Houghton, David Gray. Hodder & Stoughton Educational, 1997.

Doctors To Be by Susan Spindler. BBC Books, 1992.

See also UCAS website and bookshop (www.ucas.ac.uk) for more information and suggested reading.

Appendix 5 Website addresses for UK medical schools

These sites give up-to-date information on contacts, admissions, entry requirements, and the course structure.

Birmingham	www.bham.ac.uk
Brighton and Sussex	www.brighton.ac.uk
Bristol	www.medici.bris.ac.uk
Cambridge	www.med.cam.ac.uk
East Anglia	www.uea.ac.uk
Hull–York	www.hyms.ac.uk
Leeds	www.leeds.ac.uk
Leicester–Warwick	www.lwms.ac.uk
Liverpool	www.liv.ac.uk
Imperial College, London	www.ic.ac.uk
King's College, London (Guy's, King's, St Thomas')	www.kcl.ac.uk
Queen Mary's, London (Bart's and Royal London)	www.mds.qmw.ac.uk
St George's, London	www.sghms.ac.uk
University College, London (Royal Free and University College)	www.ucl.ac.uk/medical
Manchester	www.medicine.man.ac.uk
Newcastle	www.newcastle.ac.uk
Nottingham	www.nottingham.ac.uk/medical-school
Oxford	www.medicine.ox.ac.uk/medsch
Peninsula	www.pms.ac.uk
Sheffield	www.shef.ac.uk/-medsch
Southampton	www.som.soton.ac.uk
Aberdeen	www.aberdeen.ac.uk
Dundee	www.dundee.ac.uk/medicalschool
Edinburgh	www.med.ed.ac.uk
Glasgow	www.medicine.gla.ac.uk
St Andrew's	www.st-andrews.ac.uk
University of Wales College of Medicine, Cardiff	www.cf.ac.uk
Queen's University, Belfast	www.qub.ac.uk

In some cases the web address listed will take you directly to the medical school homepage; in others you will have to navigate your way to the medicine section, usually by clicking on courses or departments on the university homepage.

Appendix 6 Addresses of professional and specialty organisations

College of Anaesthetists, 35–43 Lincoln's Inn Fields, London WC2A 3PN.
Faculty of Public Health Medicine of the Royal Colleges of Physicians of the United Kingdom, 28 Portland Place, London W1N 4DE.

Faculty of Occupational Medicine (see Physicians).

Medical Research Council, 20 Park Crescent, London W1N 4AL.

Royal College of General Practitioners, 14 Princes Gate, London SW7 1PU.

Royal College of Obstetricians and Gynaecologists, 27 Sussex Place, London NW1 4RG.

Royal College of Pathologists, 2 Carlton House Terrace, London SW1Y 5AF.

Royal College of Paediatrics and Child Health, 11 St Andrews Place, London NW1 4LE.

Royal College of Physicians, 11 St Andrews Place, London NW1 4LE.

Royal College of Physicians of Edinburgh, 9 Queen Street, Edinburgh EH2 1JQ.

Royal College of Physicians and Surgeons of Glasgow, 234–42 St Vincent Street, Glasgow G2 5RJ.

Royal College of Psychiatrists, 17 Belgrave Square, London SW1X 8PG.

Royal College of Radiologists, 38 Portland Place, London W1N 3DG.

Royal College of Surgeons of Edinburgh, 18 Nicholson Street, Edinburgh EH8 9DW.

Royal College of Surgeons of England, 35–43 Lincoln's Inn Fields, London WC2A 3PN.

Armed forces medical services

RAMC Officer Recruiting Team, Regimental Headquarters RAMC, Royal Army Medical College, Millbank, London SW1P 4RJ.

The Medical Director General (Naval), (Attention Med P1(N)), Ministry of Defence, First Avenue House, 40–48 High Holborn, London WC1V 6HE.

Ministry of Defence MA1 (RAF), First Avenue House, 40–48 High Holborn, London WC1V 6HE.

Appendix 7 Grant making bodies for mature students

The Kate Adnams Charitable Trust (Nottingham Area). Browne Jacobson Solicitors, 44 Castle Gate, Nottingham NG1 7BJ.

Ashby Charitable Trust, R Goodwin. 7 New Street, Ledbury, Herefordshire HR8 2DX.

Lawrence Atwells Charity (Skinner's Company), The Clerk to Lawrence Atwells Charity, Skinners Hall, 8 Dowgate Hill, London EC4R 2SP.

The Blakemore Foundation, I McCauley and AF Blakemore and Son Ltd, Longacres Industrial Estate, Rosehill. Willenhall, West Midlands, WV13 2JP.

BMA Charitable Trusts, BMA House, Tavistock Square, London WC1H 9JP.

Dorothy Burns Charity, AJM Baker, Fladgate Fielder, Heron Place, 3 George Street, London W1H 6AD.

Clothworkers Company (Mary Datchelor Trust), Clothworkers Hall, Dunster Court, Mincing Lane, London EC3R 7AH.

Elizabeth Nuffield Educational Trust, 28 Bedford Square, London WC1B 3EG. (Women Only)

Foulkes Foundation Fellowships, 37 Ringwood Avenue, London N2 9NT.

Foundation of St. Mathias, The Trustees, Diocesan Church House, 23 Great George Street, Bristol BS1 5QZ.

George Drexler Foundation, PO Box 338, Granborough, Bucks HP20 2YZ.

Girls of the Realm Guild, The Secretary, 2 Watchoak, Blackham, Tunbridge Wells, Kent TN3 9TP.

Hilda Martindale Educational Trust, c/o The Registry, Royal Holloway and Bedford New College, Egham Hill, Egham, Surrey TW20 0EX. (Women Only)

PM Holt Charitable Trust, Ocean Transport and Trading Ltd, India Buildings, Liverpool L2 0RB. (Merseyside Residents Only)

Hooks Mills Educational Foundation, The Secretary, c/o Bristol Municipal Charities, Orchard Street, Bristol BS1 5EQ. (Education in Bristol)

Leathersellers Company Charitable Trust, 15 St Helen's Place, London EC3A 6DQ.

Miners' Welfare National Educational Trust, 27 Huddersfield Road, Barnsley, South Yorkshire. (Dependants of miners only)

Richard Newitt Fund (Kleinwort Benson (Trustees) Ltd), c/o University of Southampton, Finance Dept, Highfield, Southampton, Hants SO17 1BJ.

Newby Trust, The Secretary, Hill Farm, Froxfield, Nr Petersfield, Hampshire GU32 1BQ.

Royal Medical Foundation, Secretary's Office, Epsom College, Epsom, Surrey.

Royal Scottish Corporation, 37 King St, Covent Garden, London EC2E 8JS. (If born in Scotland, or at least one parent born in Scotland)

Sidney Perry Foundation, The Trustees, Atlas Assurance Co Ltd, Civic Drive, Ipswich, Suffolk IP1 2AN.

Sir Richard Stapely Educational Trust, 1 York Street, Baker Street, London W1H 1PZ.

Sir William Boreham's Foundation, The Drapers Company, The Clerk, The Drapers Hall, Throgmorton Street, London EC2.

Society for Promoting the Training of Women, Rev B Harris, Bent Lane, Warburton, Lymm, Cheshire WA13 9TQ. (Women Only)

St Marylebone Educational Foundation, c/o The Parish Administrator, St. Peter's Church, 119 Eaton Square, London SW1 9AL.

The Mercers' Company Educational Trust Fund, Mercers' Hall, Ironmonger Lane, London EC2V 8HE.

The Thomas Wall Trust, c/o WB Cook, Charterford House, 75 London Road, Headington, Oxford OX3 9AA.

William Akroyd's Foundation, Duncombe Place, York YO1 2DY. (Educated in Yorkshire)

Further details of trusts can be found in the following: *The Educational Grants Directory. The Grants Register. Directory of Grant Making Trusts.* It is especially worthwhile checking for charities in your local area.

Index

LEARNING MEDICINE